POLYMYALGIA RHEUMATICA RELIEF:
Your Personal Survival Guide

Sam Green

Copyright © 2024 Sam Green
All rights reserved.
ISBN: 9798343223361

CONTENTS

1 Introduction: my journey with Polymyalgia rheumatica 1

2 Understanding Polymyalgia Rheumatica 5

3 Getting Diagnosed: What You Need to Know 17

4 PMR and Seronegative Elderly-Onset Rheumatoid Arthritis (SEORA) 29

5 Medical Treatment for PMR 33

6 Living with PMR: Coping Strategies 47

7 Creating Your Support System 57

8 Long-Term Management and Flare-Ups 67

9 Preparing for the Future 75

10 Conclusion: You Are Not Alone 83

References 87

1 Introduction: my journey with Polymyalgia rheumatica

> *You know how you hit retirement and think you'll finally have all this time to enjoy yourself? Yeah, that didn't happen for me. Just when I thought I could relax, PMR decided to knock on my door and say, "Nope, not today!"* ~ Jasmine.

"I'm not even sure when it started exactly," Jasmine told me over coffee one afternoon. "It was this gradual thing, like a little ache here, some stiffness there. I remember thinking, 'Okay, this is what aging feels like.' Then one morning, bam—I couldn't lift my arms. It felt like someone strapped cement blocks to my shoulders overnight."

Jasmine, being her usual independent self, tried to tough it out. But things just kept getting worse. "I couldn't even get dressed without wincing. You should see me in the morning, trying to put on a pair of pants—it's like an Olympic event. Ten minutes just to get one leg in! And stairs? Forget it. I'm practically hugging the wall to get up or down, like some sort of mountain climber."

We both laughed, but I could see the toll it was taking on her. She wasn't just struggling physically—this was really wearing her down emotionally, too. "You know me," she said, "I'm always the 'glass half full' type. But lately, it feels like my cup's got a crack in it, and the optimism is just leaking out. Some days, I wake up and think, 'Is this it? Is this how things are going to be from now on?' It's draining."

POLYMYALGIA RHEUMATICA RELIEF

Jasmine's family has been a huge support, but leaning on them hasn't been easy for her. "My two girls and Joanne have been amazing. They're always checking in, helping out when I need it, but you know me—I hate feeling like a burden. I've always been the strong one, and now here I am, needing help to do the simplest things. It's not easy to accept."

But there's one place she still feels like herself: behind the wheel. "For some reason, driving doesn't hurt," she said, shaking her head in disbelief. "It's the weirdest thing. When I'm in the car, it's like my body forgets about the pain. But getting in and out of the car? That's a whole other circus act. I practically need a crane to lift me up sometimes."

The diagnosis took a while to pin down, as it often does with PMR. Jasmine went through months of tests and frustration before finally getting an answer. "I remember asking the doctor, 'So what now? Am I stuck like this?' He didn't really give me a straight answer. I get it—they don't always know. But man, you just want someone to tell you what to expect, y'know? That's the hardest part—the not knowing."

Despite all this, Jasmine's not the type to let anything keep her down for long. "I've learned to just take things day by day. I'm really choosy about who I spend time with now. I want to be around people who get it, who don't drain my energy. And even though it's tough, I'm trying to stay social. Sometimes I just want to curl up on the couch, but I push myself to get out there because I know it's good for me."

Polymyalgia Rheumatica (PMR) is one of those conditions that sneaks up on you, making simple things like getting out of bed or lifting your arms feel like moving through molasses. It's a chronic, inflammatory disorder that primarily targets the muscles in your shoulders, neck, and hips, leaving you stiff and sore, especially in the morning. While it mostly affects people over 50, anyone can feel the impact it has on day-to-day life, and the worst part? It can be tricky to diagnose, leaving many people like my friend Jasmine feeling lost and frustrated.

POLYMYALGIA RHEUMATICA RELIEF

Jasmine's experience with PMR inspired me to write this book. Watching her struggle with the sudden onset of pain and stiffness—after years of being a go-getter, always on the move—has been tough. She went from being active and social to having to plan her days around how her body felt. And as much as I've tried to help, I know how isolating it can be for her to deal with something most people don't understand.

I'm an academic researcher by trade, specializing in health sciences and mathematics, so when Jasmine was diagnosed, I immediately dove into the research. I wanted to understand what she was going through, but more than that, I wanted to see if I could help in any way—whether through understanding the condition better, finding treatments, or even just offering practical advice. But as I combed through scientific papers and clinical studies, I realized something was missing: there wasn't a lot of straightforward, relatable information for people actually living with PMR.

That's why I'm writing this book.

This isn't just about the medical facts (though we'll cover those in detail, don't worry!). It's also about real experiences—what it's like to live with PMR, how to cope with the emotional rollercoaster that comes with chronic pain, and practical advice for navigating life with this condition. It's a blend of my academic background and personal drive to support my friend, along with insights from others who've been through the same thing.

PMR is challenging, no doubt about it. But my hope is that this book will serve as a guide to understanding the condition, finding ways to manage it, and—most importantly—knowing you're not alone in this.

POLYMYALGIA RHEUMATICA RELIEF

2 Understanding Polymyalgia Rheumatica

Polymyalgia Rheumatica (PMR) is an inflammatory disorder that primarily affects older adults, causing muscle pain, stiffness, and general fatigue. It often targets larger muscle groups, such as the shoulders, neck, and hips. PMR is an autoimmune condition, meaning the body's immune system mistakenly attacks healthy tissue, which leads to inflammation. The condition can be severe and debilitating, especially in its early stages.

Key Symptoms of PMR:

1. Muscle Pain and Stiffness: The hallmark symptoms of PMR are intense pain and stiffness, particularly in the shoulders and hips. These symptoms are usually worse in the morning or after periods of inactivity. Stiffness often limits range of motion, making it difficult to perform everyday activities such as getting dressed or rising from a chair.

2. Fatigue and Malaise: Fatigue is another common symptom, often accompanied by a general feeling of being unwell. People with PMR may feel constantly tired despite getting enough rest.

3. Reduced Mobility: As the stiffness worsens, many individuals find it hard to walk or move freely. Activities that used to be simple, like climbing stairs or lifting objects, can become nearly impossible.

4. Other Symptoms: Some people with PMR also experience mild fever, loss of appetite, and weight loss, contributing to an overall feeling of illness.

POLYMYALGIA RHEUMATICA RELIEF

Jasmine's experience with PMR has been particularly challenging. It began subtly, with what she initially thought was regular muscle soreness from overexertion. But soon, her mornings became a dreaded time of day. She'd wake up feeling like her muscles had turned to stone, especially around her neck and shoulders. Getting out of bed felt like lifting a hundred-pound weight, and every movement sent a jolt of stiffness through her body.

One morning, Jasmine recalls trying to brush her hair and realizing her arms couldn't move above shoulder height without searing pain. The stiffness made basic activities—like showering, getting dressed, or even holding a cup of coffee—monumental tasks. This stiffness persisted throughout the day, but the mornings were the worst.

Jasmine also remembers a time she went grocery shopping with her son. She couldn't bend down to grab an item from a lower shelf because her hips and legs felt locked in place. It was embarrassing, and she had to ask for help. That was the moment she realized how much PMR was starting to take over her independence.

Another painful memory involves an outing with her friends. Jasmine had been determined to go hiking—a tradition she always loved. But only a short way into the trail, her shoulders and hips screamed with pain. The stiffness turned her legs into lead, and she could barely keep pace. It was the first time she felt PMR's impact not just on her body but also on her social life.

PMR is a condition that, while treatable, requires adjustments to everyday life. For many like Jasmine, it's a difficult journey of learning to manage the symptoms and their emotional toll.

Causes and Risk Factors of Polymyalgia Rheumatica (PMR)

While the exact causes of **Polymyalgia Rheumatica (PMR)** are still unknown, it's understood that the condition stems from inflammation, likely triggered by abnormal immune system activity. In PMR, the immune system attacks the body's tissues, particularly around the muscles and joints, leading to inflammation, pain, and stiffness.

This type of autoimmune activity is often linked to genetic factors, environmental triggers, or a combination of both.

Causes:

1. **Inflammation**: The root cause of the muscle pain and stiffness in PMR is inflammation, particularly in the joints and surrounding tissues. Although the exact mechanisms are unclear, inflammation in PMR is thought to be the result of an overactive immune response.

2. **Immune System Factors**: Like many autoimmune disorders, PMR involves the immune system mistakenly targeting healthy cells. Some researchers suspect that a viral infection or environmental trigger could set off the immune system's abnormal response, leading to the development of PMR. The sudden onset of PMR and symptoms such as joint pain, fever and malaise, are suspected to be a result of infections caused by viruses [1]. For example, the flu virus [2] and COVID-19 [3] have been linked to cases of PMR, but so have the flu vaccine [4] and the COVID-19 vaccination [5].

3. **Genetics**: Though not all people with PMR have a family history of the disease, there is evidence that genetic factors play a role [6]. Certain genes involved in immune system regulation are thought to increase the likelihood of developing PMR.

Risk Factors:

1. **Age**: PMR primarily affects older adults, with the average age of onset being around 70 years. It is rare for people under the age of 50 to develop the condition.

2. **Gender**: Women are two to three times more likely than men to develop PMR, although men can still be affected.

3. **Ethnicity**: PMR is more common in people of Northern European or Scandinavian descent.

4. **Weight and nutrition:** Lower BMI, green vegetable consumption, rice and olive oil all relate to lowering

the risk of developing PMR [7].

5. **Other Conditions**: People with PMR are at an increased risk of developing **giant cell arteritis** (GCA), a related inflammatory condition that affects blood vessels, particularly in the head.

Jasmine's Risk Factors:

Although Jasmine doesn't have a family history of PMR, there are still some aspects of her lifestyle that might contribute to her risk. For instance:

- **Diet and Inflammation**: Jasmine loves her red meat, and while there is no direct evidence linking a diet high in red meat to PMR, some studies suggest that diets rich in saturated fats and red meat could contribute to systemic inflammation. Diets that emphasize processed foods and red meat have been associated with higher inflammatory markers, which may worsen autoimmune conditions like PMR.

- **Overweight**: Jasmine is slightly overweight, and while weight is not a proven cause of PMR, carrying extra weight can contribute to general inflammation and make it more difficult for the body to manage autoimmune responses [8]. Obesity has been linked to higher levels of pro-inflammatory cytokines [9], which might exacerbate conditions like PMR.

- **Hydration and Health**: Jasmine doesn't drink a lot of water, and while hydration isn't directly linked to PMR, staying well-hydrated is important for joint health and managing inflammation. Dehydration can lead to muscle cramps and fatigue, which could worsen the discomfort already caused by PMR.

- **Alcohol**: Jasmine enjoys her daily glass of red wine, which contains **resveratrol**, a compound known for its anti-inflammatory properties. However, excessive alcohol consumption can promote inflammation and might contribute to the overall inflammatory burden on her body, potentially worsening her symptoms over time.

Though Jasmine's exact risk factors might be unclear, her love of red meat, tendency toward dehydration, and slight excess weight could contribute to inflammation in her body. These factors might make it harder for her immune system to regulate itself properly, leading to autoimmune flare-ups like those seen in PMR.

However, PMR remains largely an unpredictable condition, with its causes still not fully understood.

The Role of Inflammation: How Inflammation in the Body Leads to PMR Symptoms

Inflammation is at the heart of polymyalgia rheumatica (PMR). It's what makes your joints ache, your muscles stiffen, and even simple movements feel like a battle. But what exactly is inflammation, and why does it play such a key role in PMR?

At its core, inflammation is the body's natural response to injury or infection. Think of it as the immune system's alarm system. When something harmful is detected—like bacteria, viruses, or even damaged cells—your immune system activates an inflammatory response to protect you. This is usually a good thing. It helps the body heal wounds, fight off infections, and recover from illnesses. But in the case of PMR, something goes wrong.

In people with PMR, the immune system seems to go into overdrive, attacking healthy tissues for reasons that aren't fully understood. It's as if your body's defense mechanism gets confused and starts seeing your own muscles and joints as the enemy. This overreaction leads to widespread inflammation, which causes the classic PMR symptoms—stiffness, pain, and limited movement, particularly in the shoulders, neck, and hips.

Understanding the Immune System's Role

To understand how this inflammation happens, we need to look at the immune system itself. The immune system is made up of various cells and proteins that protect the body. When something triggers the immune response, white blood cells flood the affected area. They release chemicals known as cytokines, which help signal other immune cells to join the fight.

In PMR, these cytokines are released in excess. This leads to swelling and irritation in the linings of joints, as well as the surrounding muscles and tendons. Because PMR is systemic—meaning it affects the entire body—this inflammation isn't limited to one small area. It can spread throughout larger muscle groups, causing stiffness and pain in multiple regions at once.

Interestingly, PMR doesn't directly attack the muscles themselves, despite how much they hurt. Instead, inflammation affects the tissues around the muscles, such as the synovial lining in the joints and the bursae, which are small fluid-filled sacs that cushion areas like the shoulders and hips. This is why the pain and stiffness often feel worse in the morning or after long periods of inactivity—those tissues are inflamed and irritated, and it takes time for them to loosen up again.

The Vicious Cycle of Inflammation and Pain

Once inflammation starts, it can create a vicious cycle. Inflammation causes pain, and pain limits movement. Limited movement, in turn, leads to more stiffness, making the inflammation worse. It's like a feedback loop that keeps spiraling, which is why PMR symptoms can be so persistent and debilitating.

Inflammation is also closely linked to fatigue, another common symptom of PMR. The immune system is working overtime, and that takes energy. Many people with PMR report feeling exhausted even after minimal activity, a direct result of the ongoing inflammatory process. This can make day-to-day tasks feel overwhelming, contributing to the emotional toll of the disease.

Why the Shoulders, Neck, and Hips?

If you have PMR, you've likely noticed that the pain and stiffness are often concentrated in specific areas: the shoulders, neck, and hips. This isn't a coincidence. These regions have large muscle groups that are particularly prone to inflammation in PMR. The shoulders and hips are also home to some of the body's most active joints, meaning they bear a lot of strain from daily activities.

When inflammation occurs, the body prioritizes sending immune cells to these high-demand areas, which is why you often experience more severe symptoms there. Inflammation in the shoulders can also radiate down the arms, while inflammation in the hips can spread to the thighs, further amplifying discomfort.

What Triggers This Inflammatory Response?

Although the exact cause of PMR is still unknown, researchers believe that a combination of genetic predisposition and environmental factors could be to blame. Some studies suggest that certain viral infections might trigger the immune system to go into overdrive, leading to chronic inflammation. In other cases, an external factor—such as severe stress or a physical injury—might serve as the catalyst.

It's important to note, though, that while inflammation is the driving force behind PMR symptoms, it's not the root cause of the disease. The immune system's abnormal response is the underlying issue, and inflammation is just one of the symptoms of that dysfunction. But because inflammation is what leads to pain and stiffness, managing it is key to controlling PMR.

The Role of Corticosteroids in Reducing Inflammation

When it comes to treating PMR, the goal is to reduce inflammation as quickly and effectively as possible. This is where corticosteroids, such as prednisone, come into play. Corticosteroids are powerful anti-inflammatory drugs that can bring relief from PMR symptoms within days or even hours.

By dampening the immune response, corticosteroids help calm the inflammation, breaking the cycle of pain and stiffness. However, these medications don't cure PMR; they simply manage the symptoms by controlling the body's inflammatory process. For many people, corticosteroids are a lifeline, allowing them to regain mobility and improve their quality of life.

That said, long-term steroid use comes with its own set of risks, including weakened bones, weight gain, and increased susceptibility to infections. This is why doctors usually prescribe the lowest effective dose and gradually taper it down as symptoms improve. For some patients, managing the inflammatory process with steroids for several years is necessary before the condition fully goes into remission.

Targeting Inflammation Through Lifestyle Changes

Beyond medication, there are also lifestyle changes that can help reduce inflammation. A healthy diet rich in anti-inflammatory foods, such as fruits, vegetables, and omega-3 fatty acids, may provide some relief. Regular, low-impact exercise like walking or swimming can also help reduce stiffness and improve mobility by keeping the muscles active without putting too much strain on inflamed joints.

Additionally, managing stress through mindfulness practices, yoga, or meditation can be beneficial. Stress can exacerbate inflammation, so finding ways to relax and de-stress may help control PMR symptoms.

In conclusion, inflammation plays a central role in the development and persistence of PMR symptoms. It's the body's immune system gone haywire, attacking healthy tissues and causing pain, stiffness, and fatigue. While we may not fully understand what triggers this inflammatory response, controlling it through medication and lifestyle changes is essential for managing PMR and improving quality of life.

Common Misconceptions: Addressing Myths and Misunderstandings About PMR

Polymyalgia rheumatica (PMR) is often misunderstood, both by those experiencing its symptoms and even by healthcare providers. Because it shares symptoms with other conditions, and because it primarily affects older adults, PMR can be easily misinterpreted. Let's address some of the most common misconceptions that surround this illness to clear up confusion and provide a clearer understanding of the disease.

Misconception 1: PMR Is Just a Part of Aging

One of the most pervasive myths about PMR is that its symptoms—such as joint pain, stiffness, and fatigue—are simply part of the natural aging process. It's easy to see why this misconception exists, given that PMR primarily affects people over the age of 50, with most cases occurring in individuals over 70.

However, while it's true that aging can bring about certain aches and pains, PMR is not just a sign of "getting older." The severity and nature of the pain in PMR are not typical of normal aging. In fact, the pain and stiffness caused by PMR can be debilitating and life-altering, often striking suddenly and making routine daily tasks, like getting out of bed or lifting your arms, incredibly difficult. The inflammation involved in PMR is a pathological process, not just a consequence of aging joints and muscles. If you or someone you know is experiencing these kinds of symptoms, it's important to seek medical advice, as treatment can provide significant relief.

Misconception 2: PMR Only Affects the Muscles

Because PMR causes intense muscle pain and stiffness, it's easy to assume that the disease directly affects the muscles themselves. But this is a misconception. In reality, PMR does not damage the muscles directly. The root cause of the pain lies in inflammation of the tissues surrounding the muscles, such as the joints, tendons, and bursae (fluid-filled sacs that cushion the joints).

This is an important distinction because it helps explain why PMR responds so well to anti-inflammatory treatments like corticosteroids. While the muscles feel stiff and painful, the underlying problem is inflammation in these surrounding tissues, and reducing that inflammation is key to relieving the pain.

Misconception 3: PMR Is the Same as Rheumatoid Arthritis (RA)

Since both PMR and rheumatoid arthritis (RA) involve joint pain and inflammation, it's common for the two conditions to be confused. However, they are quite different in terms of their causes, symptoms, and long-term outlooks.

RA is an autoimmune disease that primarily targets the joints, leading to joint damage, deformities, and chronic pain. Over time, RA can cause permanent joint damage, which can severely affect mobility. PMR, on the other hand, does not typically cause permanent joint damage. While it does lead to joint inflammation and stiffness, PMR's hallmark is muscle pain, particularly in the shoulders, neck, and hips, rather than joint deformities.

Additionally, PMR tends to respond quickly to treatment with corticosteroids, while RA often requires more aggressive, long-term treatments such as disease-modifying antirheumatic drugs (DMARDs). Understanding this distinction is important to ensure that people with PMR receive the right diagnosis and treatment.

Misconception 4: PMR Symptoms Are the Same for Everyone

Another common misunderstanding is that everyone with PMR will experience the same symptoms in the same way. The reality is that PMR symptoms can vary greatly from person to person. While most people experience pain and stiffness in the shoulders, neck, and hips, some may have symptoms that radiate to the thighs, arms, or lower back. Others might have more mild symptoms in one area but intense pain in another.

Fatigue is also a significant symptom for many people, but the severity of this can range from moderate tiredness to debilitating exhaustion. Some individuals might also experience systemic symptoms like fever or weight loss, adding to the complexity of PMR's presentation. This variability can sometimes make PMR difficult to diagnose, particularly if the symptoms don't follow the typical pattern.

Misconception 5: PMR Will Go Away on Its Own

It's true that PMR can go into remission, but assuming it will simply go away on its own without treatment is a dangerous misconception. While some cases of PMR may improve over time, most people need medication to control the symptoms. Left untreated, PMR can cause months or even years of debilitating pain and stiffness. Moreover, untreated PMR can increase the risk of developing another serious condition called giant cell arteritis (GCA), which affects the blood vessels and can lead to permanent vision loss or stroke.

Corticosteroids are the most common treatment for PMR, and they work by quickly reducing inflammation. Without this treatment, inflammation continues unchecked, which can not only prolong symptoms but also lead to complications. While steroids come with side effects, they are usually necessary to manage PMR, and doctors will carefully monitor the dosage to minimize risks.

Misconception 6: PMR Only Affects Women

While it's true that PMR is more common in women than men—women are about twice as likely to develop the condition—men are by no means immune to PMR. It affects both genders, and men can experience the same severe pain, stiffness, and fatigue as women with the disease. This misconception can sometimes lead to delayed diagnoses in men, as they or their doctors might not initially consider PMR as a possibility. It's important for both men and women experiencing symptoms to seek a thorough evaluation, especially if the pain and stiffness seem unusual or out of proportion to normal aging.

Misconception 7: PMR Always Requires High-Dose Steroids

There is a common belief that PMR requires long-term, high-dose corticosteroids to keep symptoms at bay. While steroids are the cornerstone of treatment, the goal is to find the lowest effective dose to manage symptoms while minimizing side effects. Many people with PMR start on a higher dose of corticosteroids but are gradually tapered down to a lower maintenance dose over time. This tapering process is critical to avoid complications such as osteoporosis, weight gain, or increased risk of infections, which are more likely with long-term, high-dose steroid use.

Additionally, some newer treatments and approaches are being studied to see if they can help reduce the reliance on steroids. While steroids remain the most effective treatment currently available, ongoing research into alternative therapies may eventually change how PMR is managed.

Misconception 8: PMR Is a Life-Long Condition

Many people fear that once they're diagnosed with PMR, they'll have to deal with it for the rest of their lives. However, PMR often goes into remission after a few years, especially with proper treatment. For most people, PMR is a temporary condition that lasts between two to five years, although some cases may persist longer. The key is to manage the symptoms effectively during the active phase of the disease and work closely with healthcare providers to monitor progress.

In summary, polymyalgia rheumatica is a complex and often misunderstood condition. It's not just part of aging, and it's not the same as rheumatoid arthritis. It doesn't affect everyone the same way, and it typically requires treatment to control inflammation and prevent complications. By addressing these common misconceptions, people with PMR—and those around them—can better understand the disease and take the right steps toward managing it effectively.

3 Getting Diagnosed: What You Need to Know

Early Signs and Symptoms: What to Watch for and When to Seek Medical Help

Polymyalgia rheumatica (PMR) often begins subtly, with symptoms that might be easy to dismiss or attribute to something else, like overexertion or the normal aches and pains of aging. However, recognizing the early signs of PMR is crucial for getting prompt treatment and preventing more severe complications down the line. The tricky part is that these early symptoms can vary in intensity and might come and go before fully setting in.

Early Warning Signs

The most common early sign of PMR is morning stiffness, which tends to last more than 45 minutes [10]. This isn't your typical "I slept wrong" kind of stiffness. It can feel as though your muscles are locked in place, making it hard to get out of bed or move your arms and legs. The stiffness is often worse after periods of inactivity, such as sitting for long stretches or sleeping, and it usually affects the shoulders, neck, and hips.

Another hallmark symptom is pain. The pain can range from dull and achy to sharp and more intense, particularly in the larger muscle groups around the shoulders and hips. It's not uncommon for people to feel like they've suddenly aged overnight, with their mobility dramatically reduced. Fatigue often accompanies the pain, which can make daily activities, like getting dressed or walking, feel exhausting.

Jasmine's Experience

My friend Jasmine was a perfect example of someone who noticed early warning signs but didn't connect them to anything serious at first. She told me she started feeling unusually stiff in the mornings, but like many of us, she brushed it off. "I figured I was just getting older," she said, "or maybe it was from sitting at my desk too long." She also experienced aches in her shoulders and hips, which seemed to worsen after stressful days at work.

It wasn't until she went through a period of intense stress—juggling a demanding job, caring for her aging parents, and managing household responsibilities—that her symptoms became unbearable. Suddenly, the mild stiffness and soreness turned into constant, debilitating pain. "One morning, I could barely lift my arms to put on a jacket," she said. It was at this point that she finally sought medical advice, which led to her PMR diagnosis.

Red Flags: When to Seek Medical Help

So, when should you seek medical help? The key is to pay attention to persistent, unexplained symptoms, particularly if they interfere with your daily activities. Here are a few signs that it's time to consult a doctor:

1. **Morning Stiffness That Lasts More Than 30 Minutes**

If you're waking up stiff and sore every morning, especially if it's lasting more than half an hour, that's a red flag. While everyone feels a little stiff sometimes, this level of stiffness—especially when it's paired with muscle pain—shouldn't be ignored.

2. **Pain in the Shoulders, Neck, or Hips**

PMR typically affects the larger muscle groups in the shoulders, neck, and hips. If you're experiencing pain in these areas that doesn't seem to have a clear cause (like an injury), and it's not improving, it's worth getting checked out. The pain may start on one side of the body but can eventually spread to both.

3. **Sudden Loss of Mobility**

One of the more alarming symptoms is the sudden inability to move certain parts of your body. You may find it difficult to lift your arms above your head, bend over, or walk without pain. This kind of restricted movement isn't something to brush off, especially if it happens over a short period of time.

4. **Fatigue and General Malaise**

Feeling unusually tired, weak, or "off" can be another early sign of PMR [11]. This isn't just a little tiredness from a busy day; it's more of a chronic exhaustion that makes even simple tasks feel overwhelming. If this fatigue is accompanied by pain and stiffness, it's time to see a doctor.

5. **Low-Grade Fever or Weight Loss**

While not as common, some people with PMR also experience systemic symptoms like a low-grade fever or unexplained weight loss. These symptoms can sometimes mimic the flu, but they don't go away after a week or two, and they can signal that the body is dealing with more widespread inflammation.

Don't Wait Until It's Too Severe

Unfortunately, like Jasmine, many people don't seek medical help until their symptoms become debilitating. In her case, she spent months trying to push through the pain, thinking it would go away on its own. "I didn't realize how much I'd let it affect me until I couldn't even hold a pen to write a grocery list," she told me. By the time she saw a doctor, she was in such bad shape that immediate treatment with corticosteroids was necessary to get her symptoms under control.

Had Jasmine recognized the early signs and sought help sooner, she could have started treatment earlier, potentially avoiding the intense pain and reduced mobility she experienced. The sooner PMR is diagnosed, the sooner it can be managed, which helps prevent complications and improves quality of life.

What to Expect at a Doctor's Appointment

If you're experiencing any of these symptoms, especially a combination of stiffness, pain, and fatigue, it's essential to see your doctor for an evaluation. During the appointment, the doctor will likely ask about your symptoms in detail—when they started, how severe they are, and whether anything seems to make them better or worse.

Blood tests, such as the erythrocyte sedimentation rate (ESR) or C-reactive protein (CRP) levels, may be ordered to check for signs of inflammation. These tests aren't specific to PMR, but elevated levels can indicate that the body is dealing with an inflammatory condition. In some cases, imaging tests, like ultrasounds or MRIs, might be used to look for inflammation in the joints or surrounding tissues.

Why Early Diagnosis Matters

Getting a prompt diagnosis of PMR is crucial for several reasons. First, early treatment with corticosteroids can dramatically improve symptoms, often within days. This can restore your mobility and reduce the fatigue that PMR causes. Second, early diagnosis can help prevent the progression of symptoms, reducing the risk of long-term complications like muscle atrophy or the development of giant cell arteritis (GCA), a potentially serious condition that can affect vision and even lead to blindness if untreated.

In conclusion, PMR can be tricky to recognize in its early stages, but paying attention to persistent, unusual stiffness, pain, and fatigue is key. If you're experiencing symptoms that affect your daily life, don't wait until they become severe before seeking help. As Jasmine's story shows, catching PMR early can make all the difference in managing the condition effectively and regaining control over your life.

Tests and Diagnosis: Blood Tests, Physical Exams, and Other Diagnostic Tools Doctors Use to Identify PMR

Polymyalgia rheumatica (PMR) can be tricky to diagnose because its symptoms often mimic those of other conditions, like rheumatoid arthritis or fibromyalgia. However, there are specific tests and diagnostic tools doctors use to help confirm a PMR diagnosis. If you're experiencing symptoms like persistent morning stiffness, muscle pain, or fatigue, it's important to undergo a thorough evaluation to rule out other possibilities and pinpoint the exact cause of your discomfort.

The Diagnostic Process

Diagnosing PMR starts with a detailed medical history and physical exam. Your doctor will ask about the onset of symptoms, where the pain and stiffness are located, and how these symptoms impact your daily activities. But to confirm PMR, doctors often rely on a combination of blood tests and, in some cases, imaging studies. Each test offers valuable insight into the body's inflammation levels and can help doctors rule out other conditions with similar symptoms.

Blood Tests

Two key blood tests are often used to diagnose PMR: **erythrocyte sedimentation rate (ESR)** and **C-reactive protein (CRP)** levels. Both tests measure inflammation in the body. While elevated levels of ESR and CRP aren't exclusive to PMR, they are strong indicators of an inflammatory process at work.

- **ESR (Erythrocyte Sedimentation Rate)**: This test measures how quickly red blood cells settle at the bottom of a test tube. A faster-than-normal rate indicates that there's inflammation in the body. People with PMR typically have a high ESR.

- **CRP (C-Reactive Protein)**: CRP is a protein produced by the liver in response to inflammation. Elevated CRP levels are another sign of systemic inflammation, often present in people with PMR.

Both tests are straightforward blood draws, usually done in a lab. The results help your doctor determine whether inflammation is present and rule out other possible conditions.

Jasmine's Experience with Blood Tests

When Jasmine underwent these blood tests, she took it all in stride, as she usually does. "It's just a couple of needles," she told me, shrugging. She wasn't fazed by the process, even though she was a bit tired from dealing with her symptoms. Her results came back with elevated ESR and CRP levels, which helped guide her doctor toward a diagnosis of PMR.

Barbara's Experience with Blood Tests

Her friend, Barbara, however, had quite the opposite experience. While Barbara isn't fond of tests in general, she found the idea of blood work particularly unpleasant. "I'm not a fan of needles," Barbara said, laughing nervously. She felt anxious about the tests and admitted she was a bit uncomfortable during the process, but like many people, she knew it was a necessary step toward getting answers. Her tests showed similar inflammatory markers, but getting through the experience wasn't as easy for her as it was for Jasmine.

Physical Examination

In addition to blood tests, a physical exam is an essential part of the diagnostic process for PMR. Your doctor will likely test your range of motion and ask you to perform simple movements to gauge how much pain and stiffness you're experiencing. They may press on certain areas, such as your shoulders or hips, to check for tenderness or swelling.

During Jasmine's physical exam, she explained how the stiffness in her shoulders had become so intense that she could barely lift her arms above her head. Her doctor asked her to raise her arms, and though she struggled, this limitation was an important clue in confirming her PMR diagnosis. Physical exams like this can help doctors differentiate between PMR and other conditions that affect the muscles or joints.

Imaging Tests

While blood tests and physical exams are the primary tools for diagnosing PMR, imaging studies can also be helpful in some cases, especially when there's uncertainty about the diagnosis. Imaging tests like ultrasounds or MRIs can reveal inflammation in the joints, bursae, or surrounding tissues—areas often affected in PMR.

- **Ultrasound**: An ultrasound can help detect inflammation in the shoulder joints and hips. This test is painless and non-invasive. The doctor uses a small handheld device that sends sound waves into the body, creating images of the soft tissues and joints.

- **MRI (Magnetic Resonance Imaging)**: MRI

scans are less commonly used but can offer a more detailed view of the soft tissues around the joints. MRIs are particularly useful for ruling out other conditions, like rheumatoid arthritis, or assessing the extent of inflammation. Subacromial and subdeltoid bursitis of the shoulders and iliopectineal bursitis and hip synovitis, which are the predominant and most frequently observed lesions in active PMR, can be seen on an MRI [12]. These terms refer to inflammation of fluid-filled sacs (bursae) located near joints. Subacromial and subdeltoid bursitis occur in the shoulder, while iliopectineal bursitis and hip synovitis involve the hip joint.

Jasmine's Experience with Imaging Tests

Jasmine was recommended an ultrasound to check for inflammation in her shoulder joints. "It was simple," she said. "I just had to lie there, and they moved the little device over my skin. No big deal." For her, this test was painless, and she appreciated how it provided additional clarity for her diagnosis. Jasmine felt confident in her doctor's thorough approach, and while the ultrasound confirmed what the blood tests had already suggested, it gave her peace of mind to know everything was being thoroughly investigated.

Barbara's Experience with Imaging Tests

Barbara, on the other hand, found the idea of imaging tests more stressful. "I'm not one for hospitals or tests," she admitted. When her doctor suggested an MRI to rule out other conditions, she felt uneasy about being in the machine for an extended period. While MRIs aren't painful, the experience of lying still in a narrow tube can be uncomfortable for some people, especially those with claustrophobia or anxiety about medical procedures. Although she wasn't thrilled about the MRI, Barbara recognized its importance in getting an accurate diagnosis and braved the test.

Ruling Out Other Conditions

One of the key challenges in diagnosing PMR is distinguishing it from other conditions with similar symptoms. Rheumatoid arthritis, lupus, and fibromyalgia can all cause pain, stiffness, and fatigue, so it's essential for doctors to rule out these other possibilities.

In some cases, doctors may order additional blood tests or imaging studies to ensure there's no evidence of other autoimmune conditions. If symptoms don't fully align with PMR, they may also test for conditions like giant cell arteritis (GCA), which sometimes occurs alongside PMR. This condition affects the arteries and can cause severe headaches, jaw pain, and vision problems. If GCA is suspected, your doctor may recommend a **temporal artery biopsy**, which involves taking a small sample of the artery to check for inflammation.

Why Testing Is Important

While undergoing tests for PMR can feel daunting, as Barbara can attest, they are a necessary step in reaching a diagnosis. Without these tests, it's difficult for doctors to confirm PMR or rule out other serious conditions. Thankfully, the combination of blood tests, physical exams, and, if necessary, imaging studies provides a clear picture of what's going on in the body.

For people like Jasmine, who take everything in stride, these tests may just feel like another step in the process. But even for those who aren't comfortable with medical procedures, like Barbara, knowing that these tests are vital to getting an accurate diagnosis—and ultimately the right treatment—can make the experience more bearable.

The Importance of Early Diagnosis

Catching PMR early is crucial because the sooner it's diagnosed, the faster treatment can begin, providing relief from the pain and stiffness. Blood tests like ESR and CRP offer early indicators of inflammation, and imaging tests can help pinpoint where that inflammation is occurring. With a proper diagnosis, patients can start corticosteroid therapy, which typically brings significant relief within days to weeks.

If you or someone you know is experiencing symptoms like persistent stiffness, pain in the shoulders and hips, and fatigue, it's essential to see a doctor and go through these diagnostic tests. PMR is manageable with the right treatment, but getting to that point starts with proper testing and diagnosis.

The Role of Rheumatologists: Why Seeing a Specialist Is Key to Getting an Accurate Diagnosis in PMR

Polymyalgia rheumatica (PMR) is a complex condition, often difficult to diagnose because its symptoms can overlap with those of other diseases. Muscle pain, stiffness, and fatigue—PMR's hallmark signs—are common in several other conditions, including rheumatoid arthritis, fibromyalgia, and even common aging-related issues. That's where the expertise of a **rheumatologist** comes in. A rheumatologist is a specialist trained to diagnose and treat musculoskeletal diseases and systemic autoimmune conditions like PMR.

Why a Rheumatologist?

One of the main reasons seeing a rheumatologist is essential for PMR patients is that they are experts in recognizing subtle differences between conditions that affect the joints, muscles, and connective tissues. General practitioners (GPs) may be the first to suspect PMR, but they often refer patients to rheumatologists for confirmation because these specialists have a deeper understanding of autoimmune and inflammatory diseases.

A rheumatologist is particularly skilled at piecing together the clues presented by your medical history, physical symptoms, blood test results, and sometimes imaging studies. They can differentiate between PMR and other inflammatory or degenerative conditions that mimic it, such as:

- **Rheumatoid arthritis**: While RA can also cause joint pain and stiffness, it typically affects smaller joints and comes with more distinct joint swelling than PMR.
- **Fibromyalgia**: This condition shares some symptoms with PMR, like widespread pain and fatigue, but it doesn't involve the same levels of inflammation that PMR does.
- **Osteoarthritis**: Often confused with PMR because it also causes joint pain and stiffness, osteoarthritis is more about wear-and-tear on the joints and is unlikely to cause the systemic inflammation seen in PMR.

Rheumatologists also play a key role in ruling out conditions like **giant cell arteritis (GCA)**, which sometimes occurs alongside PMR and requires urgent treatment to prevent serious complications like vision loss.

Jasmine's Experience with a Rheumatologist

Jasmine's journey with PMR only started to make sense once she was referred to a rheumatologist. "I had been going to my regular doctor for months, but it wasn't until I saw the specialist that things really started moving," she told me. Her rheumatologist ran additional blood tests, examined her range of motion, and reviewed her symptoms in detail before confirming the PMR diagnosis. Jasmine was relieved to finally have a specialist who understood the condition and could explain what was happening in her body.

For Jasmine, seeing a rheumatologist was the turning point. The specialist's ability to identify the specific pattern of stiffness and pain, along with the inflammatory markers in her blood tests, made it clear that PMR was the culprit. "I didn't realize how much expertise was needed just to figure out what was wrong," she said.

Why You Shouldn't Delay Seeing a Rheumatologist

If you're experiencing symptoms that suggest PMR, seeing a rheumatologist sooner rather than later can make all the difference. Delays in diagnosis can mean longer periods of untreated inflammation, which not only prolongs discomfort but also increases the risk of complications, including muscle atrophy or even the development of GCA. Early intervention with the right treatment—typically corticosteroids—can reduce inflammation quickly and help restore mobility.

While general practitioners can provide an initial assessment, they may not have the specific expertise to navigate the complexities of autoimmune and inflammatory disorders like PMR. By seeing a rheumatologist, you'll get access to a specialist who knows what tests to order, what symptoms to look for, and how to tailor a treatment plan to your needs.

Barbara's Hesitancy to See a Rheumatologist

Barbara, on the other hand, was more hesitant about seeing a specialist. "I've never liked going to doctors, let alone specialists," she confessed. She initially hoped her symptoms would improve without needing to see a rheumatologist. But over time, as her pain worsened and her GP wasn't able to provide a clear diagnosis, she reluctantly agreed to the referral. Although Barbara wasn't excited about the visit, she admitted that the rheumatologist was thorough and reassuring. In her case, seeing the specialist helped confirm that she, too, was dealing with PMR, despite her initial reluctance.

The Specialist's Expertise in Managing Treatment

Once a diagnosis is confirmed, the rheumatologist's role isn't over. In fact, their expertise becomes even more valuable as they guide you through treatment. Corticosteroids, typically the first line of defense against PMR, are incredibly effective, but they need to be managed carefully. A rheumatologist knows how to find the right dosage to control inflammation without causing unnecessary side effects.

For many PMR patients, including Jasmine, the initial doses of corticosteroids bring significant relief within days, sometimes even hours. However, long-term management is essential because PMR symptoms can flare up again if the medication is tapered off too quickly. A rheumatologist carefully monitors your response to treatment, adjusting the dosage as needed to maintain balance between symptom relief and minimizing side effects like weight gain, high blood pressure, or bone loss.

In addition to corticosteroids, rheumatologists may explore other treatments, such as **non-steroidal anti-inflammatory drugs (NSAIDs)** or **disease-modifying anti-rheumatic drugs (DMARDs)**, especially if PMR symptoms persist or if there's a need to reduce steroid use due to side effects. Having a specialist who understands the intricacies of these medications and their potential interactions is key to a well-rounded treatment approach.

What to Expect from a Rheumatologist Appointment

During your first visit, a rheumatologist will likely:

POLYMYALGIA RHEUMATICA RELIEF

1. Take a Detailed Medical History

Expect questions about when your symptoms started, how they've progressed, and whether anything makes them better or worse. They'll want to know about any family history of autoimmune diseases or inflammatory conditions.

2. **Conduct a Physical Examination**

Your rheumatologist will perform a physical exam, testing your range of motion and checking for pain or stiffness in key areas like the shoulders, neck, and hips. They may press on your joints to check for swelling or tenderness.

3. **Order Additional Tests**

Blood tests like ESR and CRP are common, but a rheumatologist might also request imaging studies, such as ultrasounds or MRIs, to assess inflammation in the joints and surrounding tissues. In some cases, they may run other specialized tests to rule out conditions like rheumatoid arthritis or lupus.

4. **Discuss Treatment Options**

If a PMR diagnosis is confirmed, your rheumatologist will go over treatment options, likely starting with corticosteroids to reduce inflammation. They'll explain how the medication works, what to expect, and how they'll monitor your progress.

Trusting the Process

Seeing a specialist like a rheumatologist can feel daunting, especially if you're someone like Barbara, who doesn't enjoy medical tests or hospital visits. But trusting in the process and the expertise of a rheumatologist is critical to getting an accurate diagnosis and starting effective treatment. These specialists are your best allies in managing PMR, ensuring that you receive the right care at the right time.

In conclusion, while it may feel like just another step in an already challenging journey, seeing a rheumatologist is one of the most important things you can do if you suspect you have PMR. Their specialized knowledge can make all the difference in confirming your diagnosis, managing your treatment, and ultimately helping you regain control over your life.

4 PMR and Seronegative Elderly-Onset Rheumatoid Arthritis (SEORA)

Polymyalgia rheumatica (PMR) and seronegative elderly-onset rheumatoid arthritis (SEORA) are two of the most common inflammatory diseases affecting older adults. However, diagnosing between the two can be quite challenging, particularly in the early stages, as they share many overlapping symptoms. In fact, for a long time, PMR and SEORA were even thought to be different manifestations of the same disease, or at least closely related conditions.

Both PMR and SEORA present with joint and muscle pain, most notably in the shoulder girdle, and patients often experience significant morning stiffness, lasting longer than 45 minutes. Lab tests reveal elevated levels of inflammatory markers such as erythrocyte sedimentation rate (ESR) and C-reactive protein (CRP). Additionally, both conditions typically respond well to low doses of glucocorticoids (GCs) during early treatment. However, despite these similarities, PMR and SEORA are distinct conditions with different long-term management strategies, and correctly identifying them is essential for providing the most effective treatment.

Clinical Similarities and Initial Misdiagnosis

One of the key issues in differentiating PMR from SEORA is that both conditions can present similarly in their early stages. Muscle pain, stiffness, and elevated inflammatory markers are hallmark symptoms of both diseases. Because of this, it's not uncommon for patients to be initially diagnosed with PMR, only to have their diagnosis revised to SEORA later on. This can be frustrating and confusing for patients, as the distinction between these two diseases often only becomes clear over time, particularly as their response to long-term treatment evolves.

For example, in PMR, long-term glucocorticoid use may be necessary to control symptoms, with patients sometimes requiring steroids for several months or even years. In contrast, SEORA is often managed with disease-modifying anti-rheumatic drugs (DMARDs), and glucocorticoids are typically used only in the short term. The need for prednisone tapering in SEORA helps make the distinction clearer during follow-up treatment, but this can take time to become apparent.

Importance of Sleep Disturbances in Diagnosis

One area that is being explored as a potential diagnostic clue is sleep disturbances. Though sleep disorders are frequently reported by patients with both PMR and SEORA, they have rarely been studied in depth, especially in PMR patients. Early research suggests that assessing sleep disturbances might offer a helpful way to distinguish between the two conditions at the time of diagnosis.

A 2020 study conducted by Dr. Ciro Manzo [13] and colleagues found that patients newly diagnosed with PMR had more significant sleep disturbances compared to those with SEORA. The study showed that sleep quality was poorer in PMR patients, even before the initiation of glucocorticoid therapy. While the reasons for this difference are still speculative, it highlights the potential role that sleep assessment could play in helping doctors differentiate between these two conditions.

Factors such as mood disorders (like depression and anxiety), the duration of morning stiffness, and the levels of CRP at diagnosis were also considered in the study. These factors seem to correlate with sleep quality, providing further areas for investigation into how they might influence or reflect disease activity in PMR versus SEORA.

The Importance of Rheumatoid Factor and Antibody Testing

One of the primary tools for distinguishing between SEORA and PMR is the presence (or absence) of specific antibodies. SEORA is defined by the lack of rheumatoid factor (RF) and anti-citrullinated protein antibodies (ACPA), making it seronegative. This is in contrast to rheumatoid arthritis in younger individuals, where these markers are more commonly found. However, the absence of these antibodies can make the diagnosis less straightforward, as other conditions, including PMR, can present similarly without these serological markers. This is why physical symptoms, patient history, and response to treatment are so crucial in making a definitive diagnosis.

Follow-Up and Reevaluation

Given the difficulties in distinguishing PMR from SEORA early on, follow-up care is essential. Doctors may initially treat patients for PMR, but if the patient doesn't respond as expected to glucocorticoid therapy, a reevaluation may be necessary. Sometimes, as symptoms evolve and become more characteristic of SEORA, particularly as joint erosion or deformity develops (which is not seen in PMR), a different treatment plan is needed.

In conclusion, while PMR and SEORA share many early symptoms, they are distinct diseases that require different long-term treatment strategies. The similarities between them can lead to initial misdiagnosis, and the evolving nature of the symptoms over time often necessitates a reevaluation. Assessing sleep disturbances and monitoring the patient's response to glucocorticoid therapy over time can help clinicians make the right diagnosis, ensuring that patients receive the most appropriate care.

POLYMYALGIA RHEUMATICA RELIEF

5 Medical Treatment for PMR

First-Line Treatment: Corticosteroids

When it comes to treating polymyalgia rheumatica (PMR), corticosteroids are the first line of defense. They're often considered a game-changer, bringing swift relief to the pain and stiffness that have been nagging for months. But while corticosteroids can feel like a miracle drug for many PMR sufferers, the journey with them isn't always smooth. Let me share how this treatment affected my friends, Jasmine and Barbara, as they navigated their own experiences with these powerful medications.

Jasmine's Experience: Relief, but With Caution

When Jasmine first started on corticosteroids, she felt an almost immediate difference. "It was like someone flipped a switch," she told me. After weeks of struggling to even get out of bed in the morning because of the stiffness and pain in her shoulders and hips, suddenly she could move freely again. The relief was so dramatic that it felt unreal. "I thought, if this is what the medication can do, sign me up forever!" she joked.

But as her treatment continued, Jasmine also became cautious about her enthusiasm. The initial high doses of corticosteroids worked wonders, but her doctor explained that they couldn't be a long-term solution in such high amounts. They had to slowly reduce the dosage to avoid side effects like weight gain, high blood pressure, and other complications. Jasmine had heard the warnings about steroids causing brittle bones or making it easier to catch infections, so she was careful to follow her rheumatologist's advice.

As her dose tapered, she noticed some of the old stiffness returning, but it wasn't as bad as before. "It's like a balancing act," she said, adjusting her medication levels to control the symptoms without risking the side effects. Jasmine approached this with her usual resilience, recognizing that the benefits outweighed the risks for her, but it still required patience. She worked with her doctor to find the right dose that would keep her PMR in check without taking too much of a toll on her body.

Barbara's Experience: A Bit More Hesitant

Barbara's story is a little different. She didn't share the same instant relief that Jasmine experienced with corticosteroids. For her, it was a slower process. She was more skeptical of the medication from the start, partly because she doesn't love taking pills and partly because she had heard horror stories about the side effects. "I've never been one for medication," she said, "so the idea of long-term steroid use made me nervous."

When she finally agreed to start corticosteroids, Barbara didn't feel the immediate boost Jasmine had. Her pain did improve over time, but she had to adjust her expectations. It wasn't an overnight transformation for her, more of a gradual improvement. The stiffness in her arms and legs loosened, and she was able to move with less discomfort, but she still dealt with bouts of fatigue and had to adjust her daily routine around her new normal.

The side effects were another story. Barbara was particularly concerned about weight gain, and while she didn't experience a huge increase, she did notice her appetite changing. "I felt hungrier than usual," she admitted, and this made her extra cautious about what she ate. Her doctor worked with her to find a low dose of corticosteroids that would still manage the symptoms without pushing her into uncomfortable side effects. Barbara's relationship with corticosteroids became one of compromise—she didn't love them, but she recognized that they were helping her keep PMR under control.

What to Expect with Corticosteroids

For many people with PMR, corticosteroids are the lifeline they didn't know they needed. The way they work is relatively straightforward: they reduce inflammation in the body, which in turn relieves the pain and stiffness in the muscles. But, like Jasmine and Barbara discovered, the journey with these medications is a highly personal one. Some people, like Jasmine, feel almost instant relief, while others, like Barbara, might experience a slower, more measured response.

One thing is for sure—corticosteroids are not a cure. They're a treatment designed to manage the symptoms of PMR, often for an extended period. The trick is finding the right dose that offers relief while minimizing side effects. For some, that's a delicate balance, and it requires working closely with a doctor to adjust the dosage as needed.

For Jasmine, it was about maintaining her newfound mobility while carefully tapering the dose to avoid long-term health issues. For Barbara, it was about learning to trust the process and finding a level of comfort with medication that didn't come naturally to her.

Both had to accept that corticosteroids, while effective, are not without their challenges. But for people living with PMR, these medications offer hope, allowing them to reclaim parts of their lives they thought they might have lost to the pain and stiffness.

Managing Side Effects: Practical Tips for Dealing with the Side Effects of Long-Term Corticosteroid Use

Corticosteroids are undeniably effective for treating polymyalgia rheumatica (PMR), but they come with a catch: the side effects. Long term glucocorticoid-therapy comes with the possibility of significant side effects, including fractures, infections, diabetes, hypertension, cataracts and other problems [14].

While these medications can provide immense relief, using them over an extended period often brings unwanted changes that can feel frustrating or even overwhelming. Let's look at some practical ways to cope with the most common side effects of long-term corticosteroid use.

1. Weight Gain and Increased Appetite

One of the most well-known side effects of corticosteroids is weight gain, often caused by both fluid retention and an increased appetite. Jasmine noticed that after a few weeks on steroids, she was hungrier than usual and had to be mindful about her food choices.

What you can do:

- **Focus on Nutrient-Dense Foods:** Since corticosteroids can make you crave more food, it's important to choose healthier options. Jasmine found success in swapping out snacks for fruits, vegetables, and protein-rich foods like nuts and lean meats. These options helped her stay full longer without consuming empty calories.
- **Watch Your Salt Intake:** Corticosteroids can cause your body to retain sodium, leading to bloating and weight gain. Reducing your salt intake by cutting back on processed foods and choosing fresh ingredients can help combat this.
- **Smaller, Frequent Meals:** Barbara, who was worried about overeating, started eating smaller meals throughout the day rather than three large ones. This helped keep her appetite in check without feeling deprived.

2. Mood Swings and Emotional Changes

Jasmine was surprised when she started feeling more irritable and moody after a few months on corticosteroids. It's not uncommon for these medications to affect your emotional well-being, causing everything from mood swings to feelings of anxiety or even depression.

What you can do:

- **Practice Mindfulness and Stress Management:** Both Jasmine and Barbara benefited from mindfulness practices like meditation and yoga, which helped them manage stress and maintain emotional balance. Jasmine in particular found meditation helpful when she felt overwhelmed by the emotional roller coaster.
- **Talk to Your Doctor:** If you notice severe mood changes, don't hesitate to talk to your healthcare provider. They might be able to adjust your dose or recommend

additional treatments, such as counseling or medications to help manage anxiety or depression.

3. Osteoporosis and Bone Loss

Long-term corticosteroid use can weaken bones, increasing the risk of osteoporosis and fractures. Both Jasmine and Barbara's doctors were quick to warn them about this, and they took steps to protect their bone health.

What you can do:

- **Calcium and Vitamin D Supplements:** Taking calcium and vitamin D supplements is crucial for maintaining strong bones, especially if you're on corticosteroids for an extended period. Jasmine's doctor recommended a daily supplement, which she incorporated into her routine.
- **Weight-Bearing Exercise:** Barbara, although hesitant at first, found that light weight-bearing exercises like walking or resistance training were not only good for her bones but also helped improve her mood and overall strength. These exercises help keep bones strong by stimulating bone growth and reducing the risk of osteoporosis.
- **Bone Density Tests:** Regular bone density tests can help monitor the impact of corticosteroids on your bones. Barbara's rheumatologist recommended she get one every year to ensure they caught any potential bone loss early.

4. Increased Risk of Infections

Corticosteroids suppress your immune system, making you more vulnerable to infections. Jasmine noticed that she caught colds more frequently once she started her treatment, and she had to be extra cautious about her health.

What you can do:

- **Good Hygiene Practices:** Simple steps like washing your hands regularly, avoiding crowded places during flu season, and staying up to date on vaccinations can help reduce your risk of getting sick. Jasmine made it a point to carry hand sanitizer with her and avoid large gatherings when she knew her immune system was compromised.

- **Monitor for Signs of Infection:** Pay attention to any signs of infection, such as fever, coughing, or unusual fatigue, and report them to your doctor immediately. Barbara once developed a lingering cold, but her rheumatologist caught it early and adjusted her treatment to help her recover quickly.

5. High Blood Pressure

Steroids can cause fluid retention and affect the balance of electrolytes in your body, which may lead to high blood pressure. Barbara, already predisposed to hypertension, found that her blood pressure rose after starting corticosteroids.

What you can do:

- **Monitor Your Blood Pressure:** Regularly checking your blood pressure can help you catch any changes early. Barbara invested in a home blood pressure monitor, which she used to track her readings and shared with her doctor during appointments.
- **Exercise Regularly:** Mild exercise, such as walking or swimming, can help lower blood pressure and improve your cardiovascular health. Barbara started walking daily, which not only helped with her blood pressure but also improved her overall stamina and mood.
- **Limit Caffeine and Alcohol:** Cutting back on caffeine and alcohol can also help maintain a healthy blood pressure. Both women reduced their intake of coffee and alcohol as part of their broader health routines while on corticosteroids.

6. Sleep Disturbances

One unexpected side effect that Jasmine experienced was difficulty sleeping. Corticosteroids can make it harder to fall asleep or stay asleep, leaving you feeling tired and irritable the next day.

What you can do:

- **Create a Bedtime Routine:** Sticking to a consistent sleep schedule can help regulate your body's internal clock. Jasmine found that creating a bedtime routine—dim lighting, no screens an hour before bed, and a cup of herbal tea—made it easier for her to wind down.

- **Take Medications Early in the Day:** If possible, try taking corticosteroids earlier in the day. This can help reduce the likelihood of sleep disturbances, as the medication's stimulating effects will be less prominent by bedtime. Both Jasmine and Barbara followed this advice and noticed their sleep improved.
- **Mind Your Caffeine Intake:** Avoiding caffeine in the late afternoon or evening can also help ensure a more restful night's sleep. Barbara, who loved her afternoon coffee, made the switch to decaf after her doctor suggested it.

7. Blood Sugar Levels

Corticosteroids can raise blood sugar levels, which is especially concerning for people with diabetes or prediabetes. Jasmine, who had no prior history of blood sugar issues, was surprised when her doctor mentioned this side effect.

What you can do:

- **Monitor Blood Sugar:** If you're at risk for diabetes, it's a good idea to monitor your blood sugar levels regularly. Barbara, who has a family history of diabetes, started checking her blood sugar more frequently after beginning corticosteroids.
- **Choose Complex Carbohydrates:** Eating more complex carbohydrates, like whole grains and vegetables, can help keep your blood sugar stable. Jasmine focused on balancing her meals with protein and fiber, which helped keep her energy levels steady throughout the day.

For anyone dealing with PMR, managing the side effects of corticosteroids is part of the treatment journey. As Jasmine and Barbara learned, it's important to stay proactive, listen to your body, and communicate openly with your doctor. While corticosteroids are incredibly effective in controlling PMR symptoms, taking steps to minimize their side effects will help you feel better in the long run. Managing your diet, staying active, and monitoring any changes in your health can make a world of difference in maintaining both your quality of life and your long-term well-being

Alternative Treatments: Exploring Other Medications and Therapies That May Help

While corticosteroids are the cornerstone of polymyalgia rheumatica (PMR) treatment, not everyone responds the same way, and for some, the side effects of long-term steroid use can be difficult to manage. For Jasmine and Barbara, finding a balance between relief and side effects was a key part of their journey. But they also explored other medications and therapies to support their health alongside corticosteroids. Whether it's to reduce the steroid dose, manage symptoms better, or avoid side effects altogether, there are alternatives worth considering.

While complementary therapies like acupuncture, massage, and exercise are commonly used by patients, there is limited scientific evidence to support their effectiveness for pain reduction or improved quality of life. For example, one UK study [15] found that physiotherapy, though potentially beneficial for PMR, faces challenges due to lack of specific education and guidelines. Further research is needed to establish the efficacy and safety of these therapies for managing musculoskeletal conditions.

1. Non-Steroidal Anti-Inflammatory Drugs (NSAIDs)

In the early days of PMR, before Jasmine's diagnosis was confirmed, she tried over-the-counter NSAIDs like ibuprofen and naproxen to manage her symptoms. She found that while the medicine dulled some of the pain, they didn't address the deeper muscle stiffness or fatigue that came with her condition.

While these medications can provide short-term relief for mild inflammation and pain, they're generally not enough to control the severe inflammation of PMR on their own.

While research [16] has shown that while some patients with PMR may achieve sustained remission with NSAIDs alone, evidence for this is weak: the researchers found that NSAIDs with glucocorticoids did not shorten treatment duration or reduce daily prednisone doses compared to glucocorticoids alone. In addition, NSAIDs might cause more adverse events when used with glucocorticoids long-term. Therefore, are not usually recommended for treating PMR. NSAIDs can have various side effects, including gastrointestinal issues (e.g., stomach ulcers, bleeding), increased risk of heart problems, kidney damage, and allergic reactions. When combined with glucocorticoids, the risk of these side effects may be increased.

It's always best to consult with a healthcare professional for personalized information and advice regarding the risks and benefits of any medication.

What you can expect:
- NSAIDs can be helpful in conjunction with other treatments, especially for minor flare-ups or in the initial stages of diagnosis. However, they're not strong enough for long-term management of PMR on their own.

2. Methotrexate

For people who have trouble tapering off corticosteroids or who experience significant side effects, doctors might suggest adding methotrexate, an immune-modulating drug, to the treatment plan. Barbara's rheumatologist brought this up as an option when she struggled with the tapering process, particularly because she was wary of staying on high doses of steroids for too long. Methotrexate is often used in autoimmune diseases like rheumatoid arthritis, and in PMR, it can help reduce inflammation and allow patients to lower their steroid dose.

Barbara's experience with methotrexate: Barbara was initially hesitant about starting another medication, especially one like methotrexate, which required regular monitoring and came with its own set of side effects, such as fatigue or gastrointestinal discomfort. But her doctor reassured her that this drug could help her reduce the amount of steroids she needed to control her PMR. After starting a low dose, Barbara found that while methotrexate didn't work instantly, over time it did help stabilize her symptoms, allowing her to decrease her reliance on steroids.

What you can expect:

- Methotrexate can take several weeks to take full effect, and regular blood tests are needed to monitor for potential side effects, such as liver issues or changes in blood counts. While not everyone is a candidate for methotrexate, it can be a useful second-line treatment for those struggling with steroid management.

- While Methotrexate is associated with improved inflammatory activity and reduced prednisolone dose, it comes with a relatively high risk of adverse events [15].

3. Actemra (Tocilizumab)

One of the more recent advancements in treating PMR is the use of biologics, such as Actemra (tocilizumab). This medication works by targeting a specific pathway in the immune system (interleukin-6) that's thought to play a role in inflammation. Jasmine's rheumatologist mentioned Actemra as a potential option if her PMR became more difficult to manage in the future, especially if she had trouble tapering off steroids.

Actemra is given as an injection or through an IV infusion, and for some people with PMR, it can help reduce the need for corticosteroids. Although Jasmine didn't need this treatment in the end, it gave her peace of mind knowing there were other options if her condition worsened.

What you can expect:

- Biologics like Actemra are often considered when traditional treatments aren't enough, or when people can't tolerate steroids. Because it's a newer therapy, it's generally reserved for more severe cases or for those resistant to other medications. Further research is needed to confirm Actemra's efficacy and safety profile [17]. It's important to discuss the potential risks and benefits with your doctor.

4. Physical Therapy

In addition to medications, physical therapy can play a crucial role in managing PMR symptoms. Both Jasmine and Barbara incorporated gentle exercises into their routines to maintain flexibility and reduce stiffness. Jasmine, who had been an active person before PMR, found that guided exercises from a physical therapist helped her stay mobile, even on days when she felt fatigued. She especially benefited from stretching exercises and gentle movements that didn't strain her joints.

Barbara was a bit more reluctant to embrace physical therapy, especially since she didn't enjoy formal exercise. But her physical therapist encouraged her to try simple activities, like walking and light stretching, to keep her muscles engaged. Over time, she found that these movements helped prevent the stiffness from getting worse.

What you can expect:
- A physical therapist can tailor exercises to your specific needs, focusing on improving strength, flexibility, and range of motion. The goal is to stay active without overexerting yourself. Even simple exercises like walking, swimming, or yoga can make a big difference in managing PMR symptoms.

5. Diet and Lifestyle Changes

Research has not found a direct link between a specific diet as a prevention or cure for PMR. However, a healthy diet rich in anti-inflammatory foods may indirectly benefit PMR patients by reducing inflammation and supporting overall health [18]. More research is needed to confirm this connection. It's important to consult with a doctor for personalized dietary advice tailored to your specific needs and medical conditions.

Both Jasmine and Barbara found that making changes to their diet and lifestyle helped complement their medical treatments. While there's no specific "PMR diet," some people find that anti-inflammatory foods can help manage symptoms.

This diet should focus on incorporating plant-based foods like fruits, vegetables, legumes, nuts, and seeds, which are rich in antioxidants and fiber. Limiting sodium and sugar intake, choosing healthy fats, and staying hydrated are also recommended [19].

Specific foods that may be helpful include:

- **Fatty fish:** Salmon, tuna, and mackerel are excellent sources of omega-3 fatty acids, which have anti-inflammatory properties.
- **Fruits and vegetables:** Aim for a variety of colors to get a wide range of antioxidants. Berries, oranges, grapes, cherries, leafy greens, and tomatoes are all good choices.
- **Legumes:** Lentils, beans, and chickpeas are high in fiber and plant-based protein.
- **Nuts and seeds:** Almonds, walnuts, flaxseeds, chia seeds, and sunflower seeds are good sources of healthy fats and antioxidants.
- **Whole grains:** Brown rice, quinoa, and whole-wheat bread provide fiber and complex carbohydrates.

Jasmine, always one to explore natural approaches, started incorporating more fruits, vegetables, and omega-3-rich foods, like fish and flaxseed, into her meals. She also cut back on processed foods and sugar, which she believed helped her feel better overall.

Barbara, on the other hand, didn't make as many drastic changes to her diet but did focus on staying hydrated and eating balanced meals. While dietary changes didn't replace her medications, they gave both women a sense of control over their health and well-being.

What you can expect:

- While dietary changes won't cure PMR, focusing on a balanced, anti-inflammatory diet can help support overall health and may reduce inflammation. Avoiding processed foods, sugary drinks, and excessive alcohol can also improve your energy levels and mood.

6. Acupuncture and Massage Therapy

For some, alternative therapies like acupuncture and massage can provide relief from PMR symptoms, especially when it comes to muscle stiffness and pain. While acupuncture is often used for various pain conditions, including those related to arthritis, there is limited evidence specifically supporting its effectiveness for PMR. More research is needed to determine the benefits and risks of acupuncture for PMR patients.

Jasmine decided to try acupuncture as a way to manage the tension in her shoulders and hips. While she wasn't sure if it was making a huge difference, she appreciated the relaxing effect it had on her body and mind. Barbara didn't pursue acupuncture, but she did get regular massages, which helped ease some of her muscle soreness.

What you can expect:
- Acupuncture and massage are generally considered safe, complementary therapies. While they might not directly treat the inflammation of PMR, they can help with symptom management and improve your overall sense of well-being.

7. Mind-Body Practices: Yoga and Meditation

Jasmine found great relief in incorporating yoga and meditation into her routine. She used these mind-body practices to manage stress, which often worsened her symptoms. Gentle yoga stretches helped her improve flexibility, while meditation gave her a way to cope with the mental toll of chronic illness. Barbara, less inclined toward formal meditation, still found value in practicing deep breathing exercises to relax and stay grounded.

What you can expect:
- Mind-body practices like yoga, meditation, and breathing exercises can be powerful tools for managing stress and improving mental resilience. While they won't replace medical treatment, they can enhance your overall quality of life by helping you stay centered during the ups and downs of PMR.

Alternative treatments offer additional ways to manage PMR, giving patients options when corticosteroids alone aren't enough.

POLYMYALGIA RHEUMATICA RELIEF

Whether through complementary medications, physical therapy, or lifestyle adjustments, many people find that a combination of treatments can provide a more balanced approach to controlling symptoms and improving quality of life. Jasmine and Barbara both learned that while there's no single answer to treating PMR, exploring alternatives can open up new possibilities for feeling better.

6 Living with PMR: Coping Strategies

Managing Pain and Stiffness: Daily Tips for Reducing Discomfort

One of the most persistent challenges of living with polymyalgia rheumatica (PMR) is managing the pain and stiffness that comes with the condition. For both Jasmine and Barbara, these symptoms were a daily struggle, often worse in the morning or after periods of inactivity. However, over time, they developed simple yet effective strategies to help ease their discomfort. From gentle stretching to warm baths, here are some practical tips for managing pain and stiffness.

1. Start the Day with Gentle Stretching

The morning stiffness that comes with PMR can feel overwhelming. Jasmine would often wake up feeling like her muscles were locked in place. Instead of jumping out of bed (which she quickly learned made things worse), she started incorporating gentle stretches into her morning routine to loosen up her muscles.

Jasmine's morning stretches:

- **Neck Rolls and Shoulder Shrugs:** Jasmine would start by slowly rolling her neck in circles and shrugging her shoulders up toward her ears, releasing tension in the upper body.

- **Seated Hamstring Stretches:** Sitting on the edge of the bed, she would extend one leg at a time, reaching her hands toward her toes to stretch her hamstrings.

- **Cat-Cow Stretch:** Jasmine also found that the "cat-cow" yoga pose—a gentle spinal movement—helped loosen her lower back and hips. She did this by getting on her hands and knees and alternating between arching her back and dropping her belly toward the floor.

Stretching first thing in the morning helped Jasmine feel more mobile and ready to tackle the day, and she noticed a significant reduction in her stiffness over time.

What you can do:

- Incorporate a gentle stretching routine into your mornings. Focus on areas that tend to be most stiff, like the shoulders, hips, and back. Take it slow and avoid pushing too hard. Over time, regular stretching can improve flexibility and reduce discomfort.

2. Take Warm Baths or Showers

Warmth can be incredibly soothing for PMR-related pain and stiffness. Barbara found that taking a warm bath in the evening was one of the most effective ways to unwind and relax her tight muscles. The heat helped increase blood flow to sore areas, reducing tension and making it easier for her to fall asleep.

What you can do:

- **Warm Baths:** If possible, soak in a warm bath for 15 to 20 minutes. Adding Epsom salts, which are high in magnesium, can help further relax your muscles. This can be especially helpful after a long day or when you're feeling extra stiff.

- **Warm Showers:** If a bath isn't practical, a warm shower can still help. Let the water hit the areas that feel most tight, like your shoulders or lower back.

- **Heating Pads or Warm Compresses:** For targeted relief, use a heating pad or a warm compress on particularly sore spots. Barbara often used a heating pad on her shoulders when she didn't have time for a full bath.

3. Incorporate Low-Impact Exercise

One of the most important lessons Jasmine and Barbara learned was that staying active, even when they didn't feel like it, was essential for managing PMR. Regular movement helps maintain flexibility, improves circulation, and can actually reduce pain over time. However, it's important to choose low-impact exercises that don't put too much strain on the joints.

Jasmine's low-impact exercise routine:

- **Walking:** Jasmine started by taking short, gentle walks around her neighborhood, gradually increasing the distance as she felt more comfortable. Walking is an easy way to keep muscles engaged without overexertion.
- **Swimming:** When her joints were particularly stiff, Jasmine found swimming to be a lifesaver. The buoyancy of the water made it easier to move without putting stress on her joints. She would do simple laps or water aerobics, which helped her stay active even on bad days.
- **Tai Chi or Yoga:** Both Jasmine and Barbara incorporated tai chi and gentle yoga into their routines. These mind-body practices emphasize slow, controlled movements that stretch and strengthen muscles, improving flexibility and balance. Yoga also helped Jasmine manage stress, which often made her pain worse.

What you can do:

- **Choose low-impact exercises** like walking, swimming, or cycling. Aim to stay active most days of the week, even if it's just for 20-30 minutes. Consistency is key—regular movement can help maintain mobility and prevent further stiffness.
- **Listen to your body.** Some days may feel better than others, and that's okay. On tougher days, go easy, but try not to stop moving entirely. Gentle movement can still help, even when pain is present.

4. Practice Good Posture

POLYMYALGIA RHEUMATICA RELIEF

Barbara's rheumatologist emphasized the importance of maintaining good posture, especially when sitting for long periods. Poor posture can exacerbate muscle tension and pain, particularly in the shoulders, back, and neck. Barbara made a conscious effort to sit up straight, especially while working at her computer or watching TV.

What you can do:

- **Check your posture:** Whether you're sitting, standing, or walking, try to keep your spine straight, your shoulders relaxed, and your feet flat on the floor. Avoid slouching, as this can lead to more stiffness and pain over time.
- **Use supportive seating:** If you sit for long periods, consider using a chair with proper lumbar support or adding a cushion to support your lower back.

5. Stay Hydrated

Jasmine was surprised to learn that dehydration can actually make muscle pain and stiffness worse. After speaking with her doctor, she made a point to drink more water throughout the day, which helped her feel more energized and reduced her muscle cramping.

What you can do:

- **Drink plenty of water:** Staying hydrated is essential for muscle health and overall well-being. Aim for at least 8 cups of water a day, more if you're active or live in a warm climate.
- **Eat hydrating foods:** In addition to drinking water, include hydrating foods in your diet, like fruits and vegetables, which are naturally high in water content.

6. Rest and Pace Yourself

Managing PMR often means finding the right balance between activity and rest. Both Jasmine and Barbara learned the hard way that pushing through the pain wasn't always the best approach. On days when they felt more fatigued, they gave themselves permission to rest, knowing that overexertion could lead to setbacks.

What you can do:

- **Pace yourself:** Don't try to do too much at

once. Break tasks into smaller steps and take breaks when needed. It's important to stay active, but also to recognize when your body needs a rest.
- **Prioritize rest:** Get enough sleep each night to give your muscles a chance to recover. If you feel fatigued during the day, don't hesitate to take a short nap or rest period.

Managing the pain and stiffness of PMR can be challenging, but with the right daily habits, it's possible to reduce discomfort and maintain mobility. By incorporating gentle stretching, warm baths, low-impact exercise, and other self-care strategies into your routine, you can take control of your symptoms and improve your overall quality of life. Both Jasmine and Barbara found that small, consistent changes made a big difference in their ability to manage PMR and keep moving forward.

Sleep and Fatigue: Strategies for Improving Sleep Quality and Managing Fatigue

One of the most frustrating aspects of living with polymyalgia rheumatica (PMR) is dealing with constant fatigue and poor sleep quality. For Jasmine and Barbara, fatigue wasn't just about being tired—it was a deep, bone-weary exhaustion that often accompanied their muscle pain. Many PMR patients experience disrupted sleep because the pain and stiffness are often worse at night, making it hard to rest. Over time, the lack of restful sleep can contribute to a cycle of fatigue, making the pain feel even more unbearable. But by adjusting their daily routines and learning a few strategies, both women managed to improve their sleep and fight off some of the fatigue.

The Link Between PMR and Sleep Disturbances

The connection between PMR and poor sleep is well-documented. A study published in *BMC Musculoskeletal Disorders* found that people with PMR often experience sleep disturbances, which can be linked to nighttime pain and discomfort caused by inflammation in the muscles and joints, this poor sleep quality exacerbates fatigue, making daily activities more difficult to manage. Barbara's rheumatologist explained that when her body wasn't getting enough restorative sleep, it made the inflammation feel worse, creating a vicious cycle of pain and tiredness.

Another study highlighted in *Rheumatology International* showed that addressing sleep disturbances could have a positive impact on managing the overall symptoms of PMR . While o "magic solution," improving sleep quality is essential for anyone managing chronic pain and fatigue.

1. Establish a Consistent Sleep Routine

One of the first things Jasmine did to improve her sleep was to establish a consistent bedtime routine. Her days used to be unpredictable, and she would go to bed at different times depending on how tired she felt. This made it harder for her body to settle into a natural sleep rhythm. By committing to a regular sleep schedule—going to bed and waking up at the same time every day—she found that it became easier to fall asleep and stay asleep.

What you can do:

- **Set a consistent bedtime and wake-up time.** Try to stick to it, even on weekends. Creating a predictable schedule helps regulate your body's internal clock, making it easier to get restful sleep.

- **Create a calming pre-sleep routine.** Engage in relaxing activities before bed, like reading, taking a warm bath, or doing gentle stretches. This helps signal to your body that it's time to wind down.

2. Control Pain and Stiffness Before Bed

One of the most significant barriers to a good night's sleep for PMR patients is nighttime pain and stiffness. Both Jasmine and Barbara found that taking steps to reduce their pain before bed made a huge difference in their sleep quality. For Barbara, this meant applying heat to her shoulders and hips for 15 to 20 minutes before lying down. Jasmine took a warm bath each evening, which helped ease the muscle tension that built up throughout the day.

In addition, Barbara's rheumatologist suggested adjusting the timing of her corticosteroid medication. Because corticosteroids reduce inflammation, taking the medication in the morning and tapering throughout the day can sometimes help alleviate nighttime symptoms. It's important to talk to a doctor before adjusting any medication regimen, but this strategy worked well for Barbara.

What you can do:

- **Use heat therapy before bed.** Applying a heating pad to sore muscles or taking a warm bath can help reduce stiffness, making it easier to fall asleep. Some people also find that electric blankets provide consistent warmth throughout the night.

- **Talk to your doctor about medication timing.** Adjusting when you take medications, including corticosteroids, may help reduce nighttime pain and stiffness. This can help improve your ability to stay comfortable during the night.

3. Create an Ideal Sleep Environment

Creating a sleep environment that promotes relaxation is essential for getting a good night's rest. Jasmine found that her sleep environment was a key factor in how well she slept. She invested in a high-quality mattress that provided good support, which reduced some of the pressure on her sore muscles. She also made her bedroom as dark and quiet as possible by using blackout curtains and a white noise machine.

Barbara, on the other hand, focused on reducing distractions and keeping her room cool. Because she found herself waking up in the middle of the night feeling too warm, she made sure to keep the temperature in her bedroom on the cooler side. This helped prevent her from waking up due to discomfort.

What you can do:

- **Optimize your mattress and pillows.** A supportive mattress and comfortable pillows can make a big difference when dealing with PMR-related pain. Consider getting memory foam or an orthopedic mattress that provides even support for your body.

- **Make your room dark, cool, and quiet.** Blackout curtains, white noise machines, and keeping your room at a cool temperature (around 65°F or 18°C) can all promote better sleep quality.

4. Practice Relaxation Techniques

Stress and anxiety can make sleep even more elusive, and Jasmine found that when she was feeling overwhelmed, her pain often felt worse. Meditation and breathing exercises became a regular part of her bedtime routine, helping her relax mentally and physically before going to sleep. By focusing on her breath and clearing her mind, she was able to let go of some of the tension she carried through the day.

A research review in *Behavioral Sleep Medicine* highlighted the benefits of relaxation techniques, like mindfulness meditation, for improving sleep in people with chronic pain conditions. These practicesce the body's stress response, promoting deeper and more restful sleep.

What you can do:

- **Try mindfulness meditation or guided relaxation.** You can practice mindfulness by focusing on your breath, visualizing a peaceful place, or using guided meditation apps. Doing this before bed can help ease both mental and physical tension.

- **Practice deep breathing exercises.** Deep breathing can activate your body's relaxation response, helping you wind down before sleep. Try taking slow, deep breaths, counting to four on the inhale and exhale.

5. Manage Daytime Fatigue

Even with good sleep habits, PMR can still leave you feeling fatigued during the day. Jasmine and Barbara both found that pacing themselves and taking short naps were essential for managing their energy levels. Barbara was initially resistant to napping, but she realized that a 20-minute rest in the afternoon helped recharge her without disrupting her nighttime sleep.

Jasmine also learned to prioritize activities and delegate tasks when she was feeling particularly tired. By listening to her body and accepting that some days required more rest than others, she was able to manage her energy more effectively without feeling overwhelmed.

What you can do:

- **Take short naps.** A 15- to 30-minute nap can help recharge your energy levels without interfering with nighttime sleep. Avoid long naps, which can make it harder to sleep later.

- **Pace yourself.** On days when fatigue is particularly bad, prioritize tasks and take breaks as needed. It's important to listen to your body and not push yourself too hard.

- **Mental Health**: Dealing with the emotional challenges of chronic illness—coping with anxiety, frustration, and depression.

7 Creating Your Support System

Family and Friends: How to Communicate Your Needs and Get Support from Loved Ones

Building a robust support system is vital when navigating the challenges of polymyalgia rheumatica (PMR). The road to understanding and managing your condition can be fraught with emotional and physical hurdles, and having a solid network of family and friends can make all the difference.

1. Start with Open Communication

The first step in creating your support system is communicating your needs clearly to your loved ones. Many people may not be familiar with PMR, and they might not understand the extent of your symptoms or how they affect your daily life. Here are some strategies to facilitate open communication:

- **Educate Your Support System**: Share reliable information about PMR with your family and friends. This could be in the form of pamphlets, articles, or even links to reputable websites. When they understand the condition better, they are more likely to empathize with your experiences.

- **Express Your Feelings**: Share your thoughts and feelings openly. Let your loved ones know how PMR impacts you emotionally, physically, and socially. Whether it's frustration over chronic pain or sadness from missed social events, expressing these feelings can foster empathy and understanding.

- **Set Aside Time for Conversations**: Choose a calm, quiet time to talk with your loved ones. This allows for an uninterrupted conversation where you can express your needs without distractions. Whether it's during a family dinner or a casual coffee date, having a dedicated time to discuss your condition can help deepen understanding.

2. Clearly Outline Your Needs

Once you've opened the lines of communication, it's essential to articulate your specific needs. Consider the following aspects:

- **Physical Support**: Depending on your symptoms, you may need help with daily activities. Be clear about what tasks are challenging for you. For instance, you might need assistance with grocery shopping, cooking, or household chores. Don't hesitate to ask for specific help, whether it's running errands or simply being there to lend a hand.

- **Emotional Support**: PMR can lead to feelings of isolation and depression. Let your loved ones know when you need emotional support. This might involve simply having someone to talk to or finding a companion to attend support groups or doctor appointments with you.

- **Social Interaction**: Chronic conditions can sometimes lead to withdrawal from social activities. Communicate your desire to maintain social connections, even if you can't participate in all activities. Ask friends and family to keep you in the loop about gatherings and invite you to join when you're feeling up to it.

3. Foster Understanding and Patience

Remember that adjusting to your condition may take time for your loved ones. They may not always know how to react or what to say. Encourage them to ask questions and express their concerns. This creates a safe space for dialogue and helps everyone feel more comfortable.

- **Provide Updates**: Keep your support system

informed about your condition and any changes you experience. Regular updates can help them understand your journey better and offer support that aligns with your current needs.

- **Encourage Questions**: Let your loved ones know that it's okay to ask questions. This can help demystify your experience and facilitate a more supportive environment.

4. Seek Support Groups and Resources

In addition to your family and friends, consider joining a support group for individuals with PMR or chronic illnesses. These groups provide a platform to connect with others who understand your struggles firsthand. They can offer valuable insights, coping strategies, and emotional support that your loved ones may not be able to provide.

- **Online Communities**: Many online forums and social media groups focus on chronic illness support. These can be excellent resources for finding others who share similar experiences and can offer advice and encouragement.

- **Local Support Groups**: Check with local hospitals, community centers, or health organizations for support groups specifically for individuals with PMR. In-person interactions can foster deeper connections and provide a sense of belonging.

5. Encourage Your Loved Ones to Seek Support

It's essential for your family and friends to also find support in understanding your condition. Encourage them to talk to others who may be facing similar challenges. This could involve:

- **Family Counseling**: Sometimes, professional help can provide your family with tools and resources to understand and cope with your PMR journey.

- **Friends Sharing Their Experiences**: Encourage friends to reach out to others who might have similar experiences, fostering a more supportive community around you.

Creating a supportive network takes time and effort, but the rewards are invaluable. By effectively communicating your needs and fostering understanding among your family and friends, you can build a solid foundation of support that will empower you throughout your journey with polymyalgia rheumatica. With their help, you can navigate the challenges of PMR with resilience and grace, knowing you are not alone in this fight.

Support Groups and Online Communities: The Value of Connecting with Others Who Understand What You're Going Through

In the journey of living with PMR, the importance of connecting with others who share similar experiences cannot be overstated. Support groups and online communities provide invaluable resources and a sense of belonging that can be hard to find elsewhere. Here's why connecting with others who understand what you're going through can be a game-changer.

1. Shared Understanding and Empathy

One of the most significant advantages of support groups and online communities is the shared understanding among members. When you connect with others who have PMR, you encounter individuals who truly understand the complexities and challenges of living with this condition. They've walked the same path, faced similar struggles, and felt the same frustrations.

- **Validation**: Sharing your experiences in these settings often leads to feelings of validation. When someone responds with, "I know exactly how you feel," it can be a comforting reminder that you are not alone in your struggle. This validation helps combat feelings of isolation that may arise when dealing with a chronic illness.

- **Emotional Support**: The emotional toll of PMR can be heavy, and having a community to lean on can alleviate some of that burden. Members of support groups often share their fears, hopes, and coping strategies, fostering a nurturing environment where everyone feels supported and understood.

2. Sharing Practical Advice and Coping Strategies

Support groups and online forums are not just places for emotional support; they are also treasure troves of practical advice. Members often share their coping strategies, treatment experiences, and lifestyle changes that have worked for them. This collective knowledge can be incredibly helpful for those navigating the complexities of PMR.

- **Treatment Insights**: Many people in support groups discuss various treatments they've tried, including medications, physical therapies, and alternative approaches. This shared knowledge can help you make informed decisions about your own treatment plan.
- **Daily Living Tips**: Members often share tips for managing daily activities while dealing with PMR. Whether it's finding ways to conserve energy, adapting your workspace, or discovering new methods for relaxation, these practical insights can significantly enhance your quality of life.

3. Building Lasting Connections

Beyond the immediate benefits of advice and understanding, support groups and online communities can lead to lasting friendships. The bonds formed through shared experiences can be incredibly meaningful.

- **Long-Term Support**: Having friends who understand your condition can be a significant source of ongoing support. These friendships often extend beyond the group or online forum, creating a network of people who can celebrate your successes and help you through tough times.
- **Social Interaction**: Connecting with others who have PMR can provide opportunities for social engagement that you may otherwise miss. Whether it's a virtual coffee chat, a group outing, or simply exchanging messages of encouragement, these interactions can combat the feelings of loneliness that can accompany chronic illness.

4. Access to Resources and Information

Support groups and online communities can also provide access to valuable resources that may be hard to find on your own. Members often share links to articles, research studies, webinars, and local events related to PMR and chronic illness management.

- **Educational Materials**: Many members are eager to share helpful resources, from medical literature to personal blogs that provide insight into living well with PMR. This wealth of information can empower you to take charge of your health and well-being.
- **Event Notifications**: Many communities share information about local or virtual events, such as health fairs, workshops, and guest speakers. Attending these events can further enhance your knowledge and connect you with professionals who can provide guidance and support.

5. Finding the Right Group for You

With various support groups and online communities available, it's essential to find the right fit for your needs. Here are some tips for exploring your options:

- **Research Local Support Groups**: Many hospitals, community centers, and healthcare organizations offer support groups specifically for individuals with chronic illnesses like PMR. Look for groups that focus on your needs and preferences, whether in-person or virtual.
- **Explore Online Forums**: Websites like Facebook, Reddit, and specialized health forums host numerous groups dedicated to chronic illness support. Take your time to browse through different groups to find one that resonates with you.
- **Attend a Few Meetings**: If you find a local group or an online community that interests you, don't hesitate to attend a few meetings or participate in discussions. This will help you gauge whether the environment is supportive and welcoming.

Creating connections with others who understand the

challenges of PMR can significantly enhance your journey toward managing your condition. By actively engaging with support groups and online communities, you will not only gain practical advice and emotional support but also build a network of friends who truly get it. Remember, you don't have to navigate this journey alone—there's a community waiting to welcome you with open arms.

Working with Your Healthcare Team: Building Strong Relationships with Doctors, Therapists, and Other Healthcare Providers

Navigating the complexities of polymyalgia rheumatica (PMR) often requires a comprehensive approach that involves collaboration with various healthcare professionals. Building strong relationships with your healthcare team is essential for effective management of your condition. Here's how to cultivate these relationships to ensure you receive the best possible care.

1. Choosing the Right Healthcare Providers

The first step in creating a supportive healthcare team is selecting the right providers. Finding professionals who are not only knowledgeable about PMR but also empathetic and willing to collaborate can significantly impact your treatment journey.

- **Specialist Selection**: Typically, rheumatologists are the primary specialists who diagnose and treat PMR. When searching for a rheumatologist, consider their experience with PMR specifically. Look for reviews, ask for referrals, or seek recommendations from support groups to find a provider you can trust.

- **Integrative Approach**: Don't hesitate to include other healthcare professionals, such as physical therapists, occupational therapists, nutritionists, and mental health counselors, in your care team. An integrative approach can address various aspects of your health, including physical function, dietary needs, and emotional well-being.

2. Open and Honest Communication

Establishing effective communication with your healthcare providers is crucial for managing PMR successfully. Here are some strategies to enhance your communication:

- **Prepare for Appointments**: Before each visit, take time to jot down your questions, concerns, and any changes in your symptoms. This preparation ensures that you make the most of your appointment and can address all relevant topics.
- **Be Honest About Your Symptoms**: It's essential to communicate openly about your symptoms, including their frequency, intensity, and how they impact your daily life. Providing accurate information helps your healthcare team develop an appropriate treatment plan tailored to your needs.
- **Discuss Goals and Expectations**: Share your treatment goals with your providers. Whether it's managing pain, improving mobility, or enhancing your quality of life, having clear objectives helps your team work together effectively to meet your needs.

3. Collaborating on Treatment Plans

A successful treatment plan for PMR often requires a collaborative approach between you and your healthcare team. Here's how to ensure you're working together effectively:

- **Involve Yourself in Decision-Making**: Ask questions about the proposed treatment options and express your preferences. When you're an active participant in your care decisions, you're more likely to feel confident and satisfied with the chosen path.
- **Regularly Review and Adjust Your Plan**: PMR can be unpredictable, so it's vital to reassess your treatment plan regularly. Schedule follow-up appointments to discuss what's working, what isn't, and any new symptoms or concerns that may arise. This ongoing dialogue allows your healthcare team to make necessary adjustments to your plan.

4. Building Trust and Rapport

A trusting relationship with your healthcare providers can significantly impact your overall experience and treatment outcomes. Here are some tips to foster this trust:

- **Be Consistent and Reliable**: Attend your appointments regularly and follow through with the treatment recommendations provided. Demonstrating commitment to your health can foster mutual respect and strengthen the relationship with your healthcare team.
- **Show Appreciation**: Acknowledging your healthcare providers' efforts can go a long way. A simple thank-you or positive feedback can help build rapport and create a more collaborative atmosphere.
- **Seek Emotional Support from Your Providers**: Don't hesitate to share your emotional struggles related to PMR with your healthcare team. They can provide valuable resources and support to help you cope with the psychological aspects of your condition.

5. Advocate for Yourself

Being your own advocate is crucial when it comes to your healthcare. Here are some ways to assert yourself effectively:

- **Stay Informed**: Educate yourself about PMR, treatment options, and potential side effects of medications. The more knowledgeable you are, the better equipped you'll be to engage in meaningful discussions with your providers.
- **Don't Hesitate to Seek Second Opinions**: If you feel uncertain about your diagnosis or treatment plan, don't hesitate to seek a second opinion from another specialist. It's essential to feel confident and comfortable with your healthcare team.
- **Know Your Rights**: Familiarize yourself with your rights as a patient, including the right to access your medical records, ask questions, and receive information about your treatment options. Being aware of your rights empowers

you to advocate for your health effectively.

6. Utilizing Support Services

Many healthcare facilities offer support services that can enhance your experience and assist you in managing your condition:

- **Patient Navigators**: Some hospitals provide patient navigators who can help you coordinate care, schedule appointments, and access resources. They can serve as valuable allies in your healthcare journey.

- **Social Workers and Counselors**: Mental health professionals can provide emotional support, coping strategies, and resources for managing stress related to your condition. Don't hesitate to seek their assistance as part of your healthcare team.

By actively engaging with your healthcare team and building strong, collaborative relationships, you can significantly enhance your management of polymyalgia rheumatica. Remember, you are not alone in this journey—your healthcare providers are there to support you, and together, you can create a tailored plan that addresses your unique needs and helps you lead a fulfilling life.

8 Long-Term Management and Flare-Ups

8. Long-Term Management and Flare-Ups
What to Do During a PMR Flare-Up: How to Recognize a Flare and Steps to Manage It

Polymyalgia rheumatica (PMR) is characterized by periods of remission and flare-ups, which can be challenging and frustrating. Recognizing the signs of a flare-up and knowing how to manage it effectively is crucial for maintaining your quality of life. Here's how to identify a flare-up and steps you can take to cope with it.

1. Recognizing a PMR Flare-Up

Understanding the symptoms of a PMR flare-up is the first step in managing it effectively. Flare-ups can manifest differently for each individual, but common signs include:

- **Increased Pain and Stiffness**: One of the hallmark symptoms of a flare-up is an increase in pain and stiffness in the shoulders, neck, hips, and thighs. This discomfort may be more pronounced in the morning or after periods of inactivity.
- **Fatigue**: Many individuals experience a significant increase in fatigue during a flare. This exhaustion may not improve with rest and can make even simple tasks feel overwhelming.
- **General Malaise**: Some people report a sense

of feeling unwell or "off" during a flare-up. This can include symptoms like low-grade fever, headaches, and loss of appetite.

- **Difficulty with Movement**: You may notice increased difficulty in performing daily activities, such as climbing stairs, getting out of bed, or lifting objects. This reduced mobility can be particularly frustrating and may require adjustments to your routine.
- **Emotional Symptoms**: Flare-ups can also lead to emotional distress, including anxiety and frustration. The unpredictability of PMR may contribute to feelings of helplessness, making it essential to recognize these emotional aspects during a flare.

2. Steps to Manage a Flare-Up

Once you recognize the signs of a PMR flare-up, taking proactive steps to manage your symptoms can help you navigate this challenging time. Here are some strategies to consider:

- **Rest and Self-Care**: Prioritize rest during a flare-up. Listen to your body and give yourself permission to take a break from your usual activities. Self-care practices such as napping, gentle stretching, and relaxation techniques can help alleviate discomfort and promote healing.
- **Heat and Cold Therapy**: Both heat and cold therapies can provide relief during a flare-up. Applying a heating pad or warm compress to painful areas can help relax tight muscles, while ice packs can reduce inflammation and numb sharp pain. Experiment with both methods to see which offers you the most relief.
- **Medication Management**: If you have been prescribed corticosteroids or other medications to manage PMR, ensure you follow your healthcare provider's instructions closely. During a flare-up, you may need to adjust your medication dosage temporarily. Always consult your healthcare team before making any changes.
- **Gentle Exercise**: While it may seem

counterintuitive, gentle movement can help reduce stiffness and improve blood circulation during a flare-up. Consider engaging in low-impact activities like walking, swimming, or yoga. However, listen to your body, and avoid overexertion.

- **Mindfulness and Relaxation Techniques**: Stress can exacerbate PMR symptoms, so incorporating mindfulness practices such as meditation, deep breathing, or gentle yoga can be beneficial during a flare-up. These techniques can help calm your mind and improve your overall sense of well-being.
- **Stay Hydrated and Nourished**: Proper nutrition and hydration are crucial for managing PMR. Focus on consuming anti-inflammatory foods, such as fruits, vegetables, whole grains, and healthy fats. Drinking plenty of water can also help keep your body hydrated and support your overall health.
- **Keep a Symptom Diary**: Documenting your symptoms, medications, and activities during a flare-up can help you and your healthcare team identify patterns and triggers. This information can be invaluable in adjusting your treatment plan and preventing future flare-ups.

3. When to Seek Medical Help

While many flare-ups can be managed at home, it's essential to know when to seek medical assistance. Contact your healthcare provider if you experience:

- **Severe Pain**: If your pain becomes intolerable and does not improve with home remedies or prescribed medications, reach out to your doctor for further evaluation.
- **New Symptoms**: If you experience new symptoms that are not typical for your PMR, such as significant swelling, redness, or changes in vision, consult your healthcare team promptly.
- **Emotional Distress**: Flare-ups can take a toll on your mental health. If you find yourself feeling

overwhelmed, anxious, or depressed, consider reaching out to a mental health professional for support.

Recognizing and managing PMR flare-ups can be challenging, but understanding your body and implementing effective strategies can help you navigate these difficult periods. By prioritizing self-care, communicating openly with your healthcare team, and seeking support from loved ones and fellow PMR warriors, you can reduce the impact of flare-ups on your life and maintain your well-being throughout your journey with polymyalgia rheumatica.

Adjusting Your Lifestyle: Adapting to Life with PMR Over Time—Finding New Routines and Self-Care Practices

Living with polymyalgia rheumatica (PMR) often requires significant adjustments to your daily life and routines. As you navigate the complexities of this chronic condition, finding new ways to adapt and prioritize self-care is essential for your overall well-being. Here are some strategies for adjusting your lifestyle to accommodate your journey with PMR.

1. Embracing Flexibility in Your Routine

One of the most important lessons you'll learn as you live with PMR is the value of flexibility. Your symptoms may fluctuate from day to day, so it's crucial to develop a routine that allows for adaptability.

- **Create a Daily Schedule**: Establish a daily routine that includes time for self-care, physical activity, and rest. However, be open to adjusting this schedule based on how you feel. If you wake up with increased pain or fatigue, don't hesitate to modify your plans and prioritize rest.
- **Prioritize Tasks**: Consider using a priority system for daily tasks. Identify which activities are essential and focus on completing those first. If you find yourself running low on energy, it's okay to defer non-urgent tasks to another day.

2. Incorporating Self-Care Practices

Self-care is more than just a buzzword; it's a critical component of managing PMR effectively. Developing a personalized self-care routine can help you cope with the physical and emotional challenges of the condition.

- **Mindfulness and Stress Reduction**: Practicing mindfulness through meditation, deep breathing, or gentle yoga can significantly impact your mental well-being. Set aside time each day to engage in mindfulness practices that resonate with you, helping to reduce stress and promote relaxation.
- **Physical Activity**: Regular, low-impact exercise is essential for maintaining mobility and overall health. Activities such as walking, swimming, and tai chi can help keep your body active without exacerbating your symptoms. Listen to your body and adjust the intensity and duration of your workouts as needed.
- **Nutrition and Hydration**: A balanced diet plays a crucial role in managing PMR. Focus on consuming anti-inflammatory foods, such as leafy greens, berries, nuts, and fatty fish, while staying hydrated throughout the day. Consider consulting with a nutritionist to develop a meal plan tailored to your needs.

3. Seeking Balance Between Activity and Rest

Striking a balance between activity and rest is vital for managing PMR. Overexertion can lead to increased symptoms, while excessive rest can contribute to stiffness and decreased mobility.

- **Implement Rest Periods**: Incorporate regular breaks into your day, especially during physically demanding activities. Short rest periods can help recharge your energy and reduce fatigue. Listen to your body's signals, and don't hesitate to take a break when needed.
- **Engage in Gentle Movement**: Even on days when you're experiencing fatigue, gentle movements such as stretching or light yoga can help alleviate stiffness and maintain flexibility. Aim for short sessions of movement to keep your body engaged without overexerting yourself.

4. Finding Supportive Activities and Hobbies

Engaging in activities and hobbies that bring you joy can significantly enhance your emotional well-being. Finding new pursuits or rediscovering old interests can provide a sense of purpose and fulfillment.

- **Explore Creative Outlets**: Consider taking up creative hobbies such as painting, knitting, or writing. These activities can be therapeutic and serve as a distraction from pain and discomfort.
- **Connect with Nature**: Spending time outdoors can improve your mood and overall well-being. Whether it's a leisurely walk in the park or gardening, connecting with nature can be revitalizing and grounding.

5. Building a Strong Support Network

As you adjust your lifestyle, it's essential to surround yourself with a supportive network of friends and family. Leaning on your loved ones can provide emotional support and practical assistance as you navigate life with PMR.

- **Communicate Your Needs**: Don't hesitate to express your needs to your support network. Let them know how they can help, whether it's running errands, providing companionship, or simply being there to listen.
- **Engage in Shared Activities**: Involve your loved ones in activities you enjoy, whether it's cooking a meal together, attending a class, or going for a walk. Shared experiences can strengthen your relationships and provide much-needed encouragement.

6. Accepting Change and Progress

Adjusting to life with PMR is an ongoing process that may involve ups and downs. Embrace the changes that come with your journey and recognize that progress may take time.

- **Practice Self-Compassion**: Be gentle with yourself as you adapt to new routines and self-care practices. Acknowledge that it's okay to have difficult days and that your worth is not defined by your ability to accomplish tasks.

- **Celebrate Small Wins**: Take time to celebrate your achievements, no matter how small they may seem. Whether it's completing a task you thought was too challenging or successfully incorporating a new self-care practice, recognizing your progress can boost your motivation.

Adjusting your lifestyle to accommodate PMR is a journey that requires patience, resilience, and self-awareness. By embracing flexibility, prioritizing self-care, and seeking support, you can cultivate a fulfilling life despite the challenges of living with polymyalgia rheumatica. Remember, you are not alone on this journey, and with time, you can find ways to thrive and live well with PMR.

9 Preparing for the Future

Remission and Relapse: What to Expect When PMR Goes into Remission and How to Handle Relapses

Living with polymyalgia rheumatica (PMR) can often feel like a roller coaster ride, marked by unpredictable swings between periods of remission and the challenges of relapse. Understanding these phases is crucial for managing your condition and preparing for the future. Here's what to expect when PMR goes into remission, along with strategies to handle relapses effectively.

1. Understanding Remission

Remission in PMR refers to a period when symptoms significantly improve or completely disappear, allowing individuals to regain a sense of normalcy in their daily lives. This phase can be both a relief and a source of hope, but it also comes with its own considerations.

- **Recognizing Remission**: During remission, you may notice a reduction in pain, stiffness, and fatigue. Daily activities become more manageable, and you may feel more energetic and capable of engaging in social interactions or hobbies that you previously found challenging.
- **Monitoring Your Condition**: Even when in remission, it's important to continue monitoring your symptoms and overall health. Keep regular appointments with your healthcare provider to discuss any changes and ensure that your treatment plan remains effective.

- **Staying Proactive**: Use this period to establish healthy habits that can help maintain your well-being. Focus on nutrition, gentle exercise, stress management, and self-care practices that support your overall health.

2. Planning for Future Activities

A period of remission offers a valuable opportunity to plan activities and set goals that may have felt unattainable during flare-ups. Here are some tips to help you make the most of this time:

- **Set Realistic Goals**: While it's tempting to dive back into all the activities you missed during flares, set realistic and achievable goals. Break larger tasks into smaller, manageable steps to avoid overwhelming yourself.
- **Communicate with Loved Ones**: Share your plans and goals with friends and family. Their support can help you stay accountable and provide encouragement as you engage in activities you enjoy.
- **Maintain Flexibility**: Understand that while you may be feeling better, PMR can be unpredictable. Remain flexible in your plans and be prepared to adjust them if your symptoms change.

3. Understanding Relapse

A relapse refers to the return of PMR symptoms after a period of improvement or remission. This can be disheartening, but understanding the nature of relapses can help you navigate this challenging time.

- **Recognizing Triggers**: While the exact cause of relapses can be elusive, some common triggers include stress, illness, or changes in your routine. Keeping a symptom diary can help identify patterns and potential triggers that may lead to a relapse.
- **Accepting Emotional Responses**: Experiencing a relapse can evoke a range of emotions, including frustration, sadness, and anxiety. It's essential to acknowledge these feelings and allow yourself the space to process them.

4. Strategies for Managing Relapses

When faced with a relapse, taking proactive steps can help you manage your symptoms effectively and regain control of your health.

- **Reassess Your Treatment Plan**: If you notice a return of symptoms, consult your healthcare provider to discuss your current treatment plan. They may recommend adjustments to your medication or explore additional therapies that can help alleviate your symptoms.
- **Implement Self-Care Strategies**: Prioritize self-care during a relapse. Focus on rest, hydration, and nutrition, and consider gentle activities such as stretching or light walking to maintain mobility without overexerting yourself.
- **Utilize Support Systems**: Don't hesitate to lean on your support system during a relapse. Communicate with friends and family about what you're experiencing and how they can assist you. Consider reaching out to support groups or online communities for additional encouragement and shared experiences.
- **Practice Mindfulness and Stress Management**: High levels of stress can exacerbate PMR symptoms. Incorporate mindfulness practices, such as meditation or deep breathing exercises, to help manage stress and promote relaxation during a relapse.

5. Moving Forward with Hope

While relapses can be discouraging, it's important to remember that they are often temporary. Focusing on self-compassion and resilience can help you navigate these challenging moments and maintain hope for the future.

- **Celebrate Progress**: Reflect on the progress you made during your remission phase and celebrate the small victories, even during a relapse. Recognizing your achievements can provide motivation and encourage a positive outlook.
- **Stay Informed and Empowered**: Continue

educating yourself about PMR, its management, and emerging research. Knowledge is empowering, and staying informed can help you feel more in control of your health journey.

- **Embrace the Journey**: Living with PMR is a unique journey, filled with ups and downs. Embrace the lessons learned during both remission and relapse phases, and use these experiences to foster resilience and strength as you prepare for the future.

Understanding the dynamics of remission and relapse is crucial for effectively managing PMR. By being proactive, utilizing support systems, and embracing a positive mindset, you can navigate these fluctuations with grace and resilience. Remember, every journey has its challenges, but with determination and the right support, you can thrive even in the face of adversity.

Aging with PMR: Managing the Condition as You Age and Ensuring Long-Term Health

As you navigate the complexities of living with polymyalgia rheumatica (PMR), it's essential to consider the unique challenges that may arise as you age. The interplay between aging and chronic conditions like PMR can affect your overall health, well-being, and quality of life. By understanding these dynamics and proactively managing your health, you can foster a fulfilling and vibrant life well into your later years.

1. Understanding the Impact of Aging on PMR

Aging can influence PMR in several ways, both physically and emotionally. As you age, it's important to recognize the following factors:

- **Changes in Muscle and Joint Health**: With aging, there can be a natural decline in muscle mass and joint function. This can exacerbate the symptoms of PMR, leading to increased stiffness and decreased mobility. Being aware of these changes can help you implement strategies to counteract them.

- **Increased Risk of Comorbidities**: Older adults often face a higher risk of developing other chronic conditions, such as arthritis, cardiovascular disease, or osteoporosis. Managing PMR alongside these conditions may require a more comprehensive approach to your healthcare.

- **Cognitive and Emotional Health**: Aging can bring about cognitive changes, and chronic conditions like PMR may contribute to emotional challenges, including depression or anxiety. Prioritizing mental health and emotional well-being is crucial as you age.

2. Strategies for Managing PMR as You Age

To ensure long-term health while living with PMR, consider the following strategies that promote a proactive and holistic approach to your well-being:

- **Stay Active**: Regular physical activity is vital for maintaining strength, flexibility, and overall health as you age. Engage in low-impact exercises, such as walking, swimming, tai chi, or yoga, which can help improve mobility without putting excessive strain on your joints. Aim for at least 150 minutes of moderate aerobic activity each week, coupled with muscle-strengthening exercises on two or more days.

- **Prioritize Nutrition**: A balanced and nutritious diet is essential for supporting your health as you age. Focus on consuming a variety of whole foods, including fruits, vegetables, lean proteins, whole grains, and healthy fats. Consider consulting with a registered dietitian who can help you develop a meal plan that addresses your specific nutritional needs and supports your PMR management.

- **Maintain Regular Check-Ups**: Schedule regular appointments with your healthcare team to monitor your PMR and address any emerging health concerns. Regular check-ups allow for early detection and intervention, which can be crucial for managing both PMR and any age-related health issues.

- **Manage Medications Carefully**: As you age, you may find yourself taking multiple medications for various conditions. It's important to work closely with your healthcare provider to ensure that your medications for PMR and any other health issues do not interact negatively. Regularly review your medication regimen and discuss any concerns with your doctor.

3. Fostering Emotional and Mental Well-Being

Maintaining emotional and mental health is particularly important as you age with PMR. Here are some strategies to support your well-being:

- **Engage in Social Activities**: Stay socially active by participating in community groups, classes, or clubs that interest you. Social connections can provide emotional support, reduce feelings of isolation, and enhance your overall quality of life.
- **Practice Mindfulness and Stress Reduction**: Incorporating mindfulness practices, such as meditation or gentle yoga, can help reduce stress and promote mental clarity. Mindfulness encourages you to be present in the moment and can improve your emotional resilience in the face of challenges.
- **Seek Professional Support**: If you find yourself struggling with emotional distress or mental health concerns, consider seeking support from a mental health professional. Therapy or counseling can provide valuable coping strategies and a safe space to express your feelings.

4. Creating a Supportive Environment

As you age, creating a supportive home environment can help you manage PMR more effectively:

- **Make Modifications for Accessibility**: Consider making adjustments to your living space to enhance accessibility. This may include installing grab bars in the bathroom, using a shower chair, or rearranging furniture to create clear pathways.
- **Utilize Assistive Devices**: Explore the use of assistive devices, such as walking aids or reachers, to help

maintain independence and ease daily tasks. These tools can enhance your mobility and prevent falls, which can be especially important as you age.

- **Build a Care Team**: Engage your family and friends in your healthcare journey. Having a network of support can help you navigate the challenges of aging with PMR. Discuss your needs with loved ones and encourage them to be involved in your health management.

5. Embracing a Positive Outlook

While aging with PMR presents its challenges, maintaining a positive outlook and a proactive mindset can greatly enhance your quality of life. Here are some tips to cultivate optimism and resilience:

- **Focus on What You Can Control**: While you may not be able to change your condition, you can control how you respond to it. Focus on setting achievable goals and celebrate your progress, no matter how small.

- **Practice Gratitude**: Incorporate a gratitude practice into your daily routine. Reflect on the things you appreciate, whether it's the support of loved ones, moments of joy, or small accomplishments. Gratitude can shift your perspective and foster a more positive mindset.

- **Stay Engaged with Life**: Pursue activities that bring you joy and fulfillment, whether it's a hobby, volunteering, or spending time with loved ones. Staying engaged with life can boost your mood and enhance your overall well-being.

Aging with PMR is a journey that requires resilience, adaptability, and a proactive approach to health. By implementing strategies for physical, emotional, and mental well-being, you can navigate the challenges of PMR and embrace a vibrant life as you age. Remember, your journey is unique, and with the right support and resources, you can thrive in the face of adversity.

10 Conclusion: You Are Not Alone

As we reach the end of this journey together, I want to take a moment to reflect on everything we've discussed and share some final thoughts. Living with polymyalgia rheumatica (PMR) can feel isolating, and it's easy to succumb to feelings of despair and uncertainty. However, it's vital to remember that you are not alone. There is a whole community of individuals who understand your struggles and are walking this path alongside you.

Final Thoughts

The road with PMR can be winding and unpredictable, filled with moments of hope and setbacks alike. It's a condition that can challenge your physical and emotional well-being, but it does not define who you are. Embrace your resilience; you have navigated the complexities of this disease with courage and tenacity.

As you move forward, consider the following reminders:

- **Empower Yourself**: Knowledge is your greatest ally. The more you understand PMR, its symptoms, and its management strategies, the more empowered you become to take control of your health. Advocate for yourself in healthcare settings and remain an active participant in your treatment plan.
- **Connect with Others**: Share your experiences and connect with fellow PMR patients. Hearing their stories and offering support can foster a sense of community and

belonging. Together, you can find encouragement and hope, reminding one another that no one has to face this journey alone.

- **Prioritize Self-Care**: Your health is your priority. Make self-care an integral part of your daily routine. Whether it's through exercise, mindfulness, or simply taking time to relax, nurturing your body and mind will serve you well on this journey.
- **Embrace Change**: Accept that living with PMR may require adjustments to your lifestyle. Embrace these changes as opportunities for growth and self-discovery. Whether it's finding new hobbies that accommodate your physical abilities or reevaluating your priorities, be open to the evolution of your journey.
- **Celebrate Small Victories**: Every step forward, no matter how small, is a victory. Celebrate your accomplishments, whether it's managing a challenging symptom or engaging in an activity you love. These moments of joy can uplift your spirit and motivate you to keep pushing forward.

Resources

To support you as you navigate life with PMR, I've compiled a list of helpful resources. These include books, websites, and support groups where you can find information, community, and encouragement.

Books

1. **"The Autoimmune Solution" by Dr. Amy Myers**

A guide that explores the link between autoimmune diseases and lifestyle choices, offering strategies for healing through diet and nutrition.

2. **"The FibroManual: A Complete Fibromyalgia Treatment Guide for You and Your Doctor" by Dr. Ginevra Liptan**

While focused on fibromyalgia, this book provides valuable

insights into managing chronic pain and fatigue that may resonate with PMR patients.

    3.   **"Healing the Gut" by Dr. John T. D'Adamo**

An exploration of how gut health impacts overall wellness, offering practical tips for maintaining a healthy digestive system.

Websites

    1.   **The Arthritis Foundation**

www.arthritis.org

A comprehensive resource for information on various forms of arthritis and related conditions, including PMR.

    2.   **The National Institutes of Health (NIH)**

www.nih.gov

A wealth of research-based information on PMR and autoimmune diseases, including the latest studies and treatment options.

    3.   **The Mayo Clinic**

www.mayoclinic.org

Provides reliable information on PMR symptoms, causes, treatment options, and lifestyle management.

Support Groups

    1.   **The PMR Support Group on Facebook**

An active online community where individuals living with PMR share experiences, advice, and support.

    2.   **The Arthritis Foundation Support Groups**

Find local support groups through the Arthritis Foundation's website, connecting you with others in your area who understand your journey.

    3.   **Meetup.com**

Search for local PMR or autoimmune disease support groups on Meetup to connect with others face-to-face in your community.

In Closing

As you continue on this path, know that every step you take is a testament to your strength and resilience. The journey with PMR is undoubtedly challenging, but with the right support and resources, you can navigate it with confidence and grace.

Remember, you are not alone. There is a community that stands with you, a wealth of knowledge at your fingertips, and a future filled with potential waiting to be discovered. Embrace each day as an opportunity to grow, learn, and connect. The challenges of PMR may shape your life, but they do not define it.

References

1. Cimmino MA. Genetic and environmental factors in polymyalgia rheumatica. *Ann Rheum Dis.* 1997; **56**: 576–7.

2. Duhaut P, Bosshard S, Dumontet C. Giant cell arteritis and polymyalgia rheumatica: role of viral infections. Clin Exp Rheumatol. 2000 Jul-Aug;18(4 Suppl 20):S22-3. PMID: 10948753.

3. Duarte-Salazar C, Vazquez-Meraz JE, Ventura-Ríos L, Hernández-Díaz C, Arellano-Galindo J. Polymyalgia Rheumatica Post-SARS-CoV-2 Infection. Case Reports Immunol. 2024 Mar 14;2024:6662652. doi: 10.1155/2024/6662652. PMID: 38516555; PMCID: PMC10957256.

4. Liozon E, Parreau S, Filloux M, Dumonteil S, Gondran G, Bezanahary H, et al. Giant cell arteritis or polymyalgia rheumatica after influenza vaccination: a study of 12 patients and a literature review. *Autoimmun Rev.* 2021; **20**:102732.

5. 16Mettler C, Jonville-Bera A-P, Grandvuillemin A, Treluyer J-M, Terrier B, Chouchana L. Risk of giant cell arteritis and polymyalgia rheumatica following COVID-19 vaccination: a global pharmacovigilance study. Rheumatology (Oxford). 2022; 61: 865–7.

6. Guillermo Carvajal Alegria, Sara Boukhlal, Divi Cornec, Valérie Devauchelle-Pensec, The pathophysiology of polymyalgia rheumatica, small pieces of a big puzzle, Autoimmunity Reviews, Volume 19, Issue 11, 2020, 102670, ISSN 1568-9972, https://doi.org/10.1016/j.autrev.2020.102670.(https://www.sciencedirect.com/science/article/pii/S1568997222030245 7)

7. Kulakli, F., & Caglayan, G. (2021). Nutrition and stress: Two important external factors in polymyalgia rheumatica . *Annals of Medical Research*, *28*(2), 0438–0444. Retrieved from https://annalsmedres.org/index.php/aomr/article/view/367

8. Scott, I. et al. THE RELATIONSHIP BETWEEN OBESITY AND OUTCOMES IN PATIENTS WITH POLYMYALGIA RHEUMATICA. Oral Presentation. Downloaded from https://academic.oup.com/rheumatology/article/59/Supplement_2/keaa110.037/5822295 on 14 October 2024

9. Meysam Moghbeli, Hamed Khedmatgozar, Mehran Yadegari, Amir Avan, Gordon A. Ferns, Majid Ghayour Mobarhan, Chapter Five - Cytokines and the immune response in obesity-related disorders, Editor(s): Gregory S. Makowski,Advances in Clinical Chemistry, Elsevier, Volume 101, 2021, Pages 135-168, ISSN 0065-2423, ISBN 9780128244159, https://doi.org/10.1016/bs.acc.2020.06.004.
(https://www.sciencedirect.com/science/article/pii/S0065242320300767)

10. Manzo, C. et al. Not just pain and morning stiffness duration in the daily experience of patients with polymyalgia rheumatica. Does the rheumatologist listen to all patient-reported outcomes? Reumatologia 2021; 59, 3: 200–202 DOI: https://doi.org/10.5114/reum.2021.106221

11. Green, D., Muller, S., Mallen, C., & Hider, S. (2014). Fatigue as a precursor to polymyalgia rheumatica: an explorative retrospective cohort study. *Scandinavian Journal of Rheumatology*, *44*(3), 219–223. https://doi.org/10.3109/03009742.2014.959047

12. Pavlica, P. et al. Magnetic resonance imaging in the diagnosis of PMR. Clin Exp Rheumatol 2000; 18 (Suppl. 29): S38-S39

13. Manzo, C. Subjective sleep disturbances at the time of diagnosis in patients with polymyalgia rheumatica and in patients with seronegative elderly-onset rheumatoid arthritis. A pilot study. Reumatologia 2020; 58, 4: 196–201 DOI: https://doi.org/10.5114/reum.2020.98430

14. Spies et al. Methotrexate treatment in large vessel vasculitis and polymyalgia rheumatica. Clin Exp Rheumatol 2010; 28 (Suppl. 61): S172-S177.

15. O'Brien, A. V. (2023). The role of physiotherapy in polymyalgia rheumatica in the United Kingdom: a mixed method study. (Thesis). Keele University. Retrieved from https://keele-repository.worktribe.com/output/674475

16. Hernández-Rodríguez J, Cid MC, López-Soto A, Espigol-Frigolé G, Bosch X. Treatment of Polymyalgia Rheumatica: A Systematic Review. *Arch Intern Med.* 2009;169(20):1839–1850. doi:10.1001/archinternmed.2009.352

17. Devauchelle-Pensec V, Carvajal-Alegria G, Dernis E, et al. Effect of Tocilizumab on Disease Activity in Patients With Active Polymyalgia Rheumatica Receiving Glucocorticoid Therapy: A Randomized Clinical Trial. *JAMA.* 2022;328(11):1053–1062. doi:10.1001/jama.2022.15459

18. Kulakli , F. Diet and Stress: A Case Report and Review of the Literature. Eurasian Journal of Medicine and Oncology. DOI: 10.14744/ejmo.2018.0064

19. Winderl, A. Which Foods Might Help With Polymyalgia Rheumatica? An anti-inflammatory diet is your best bet when coping with this painful autoimmune condition.

POLYMYALGIA RHEUMATICA RELIEF

https://www.healthcentral.com/condition/polymyalgia-rheumatica/diet-for-polymyalgia-rheumatica

Printed in Great Britain
by Amazon